Contents

Colour plate section falls after page 122

Foreword

There are few things more frightening than losing your sight, whether suddenly, as a result of an accident or a malignant growth, or slowly, through retinopathy or a cataract. However knowledgeable the patient is, however clearly the surgeon explains your prognosis, there remains this fear that you will be visually impaired for the rest of your life.

And, at this point in time, there is nothing more reassuring than finding yourself in the hands of a competent, knowledgeable and empathic nurse who not only understands how you feel, but is skilled enough to help you adapt to the treatment and life change demands and who can help you move forward.

There is no doubt that the nurse will be familiar with Stollery and will use it as her first choice for clinical professional updating. Written by those best of teachers; lecturer practitioners who in their day-to-day work constantly practice nursing informed by the most up-to-date knowledge available. Lecturer practitioners understand the linking of theory with practice and how that blend informs the delivery of skilled and compassionate nursing care.

There is no doubt that this text is excellent, well written, patient focused and able to clearly explain the complexities of the wide range of ophthalmic conditions.

It forms a valuable resource not just for those working in ophthalmic units but also as a reference for the many staff who work with older people, the diabetic patient, the middle aged man with spondylitis, and the practice nurse. All these need to not only understand ophthalmic treatments but need to explain them to patients and carers. It is these nurses who will ensure the glaucoma patients understand the need for total compliance in the installation of their drops; it is these nurses who appreciate patient education may mean the diabetic doesn't get retinopathy and it is the nurse in the nursing home who will recognise the signs of early cataract and ensure consultation and treatment.

In the preface Mary Shaw and Agnes Lee write of the many changes that have taken place in ophthalmology and ophthalmic nursing since the first edition was published some twenty years ago. Ophthalmic nurses have expanded their roles, providing almost the total interventions for those with chronic conditions and taking on an increasing number of tasks which were once the remit of ophthalmologists.

But for all this change, all this advancement of role, and skill, and practice, the fundamentals of all that is best in nursing still lies in the hands of ophthalmic nurses who care for patients who face, albeit hopefully temporarily, one of the greatest fears known to man.

This book will help them achieve that high level of knowledgeable practice which serves patients best.

Betty Kershaw DBE FRCN

Preface

Since 1997, ophthalmic nursing and ophthalmic care practices have moved on in leaps and bounds.

There have been several reasons for this including the government targets to bring down hospital waiting times, new approaches to patient management with a move away from inpatient care to mainly day case management and primary care settings. Ophthalmic nursing has been transformed by the involvement of others in ophthalmic nursing care such as clinical support workers, assistant practitioners and surgical care assistants. In the UK there are now several ophthalmic nurse consultants and they are at the vanguard of change. Ophthalmic nurses have become more skilled and knowledgeable within their speciality. Many ophthalmic nurses have focussed on a particular area interest to advance their practice, in many instances taking on a clinical caseload. This has included their taking on board more duties and responsibilities previously undertaken by medical staff.

Those involved in ophthalmic care have long looked to 'Stollery' to help and guide their practice. In editing this edition we have merely sought to build on the framework that has stood the test of time. Newer source materials have been included and are reflected in each chapter. Within the References and Further Reading list are recommendations for reading, including accessing the Web. These texts should help the nurse new to ophthalmic care as well as the busy practicing ophthalmic nurse.

For the sake of ease and clarity, the nurse is referred to as 'she' and the patient as 'he' with no discrimination intended.

Mary Shaw and Agnes Lee

Acknowledgements

We would like to thank our families, friends and colleagues who have helped us write this edition.

We are especially grateful to staff at the Manchester Royal Eye Hospital and The University of Manchester for their encouragement. Special thanks go to the staff in the ophthalmic imaging department at the Manchester Royal Eye Hospital, for permission to use the colour photographs. We are deeply indebted to all of the secretaries for their patience and assistance with our repeated requests for advice.

This book is dedicated to those in our families who sadly died whilst we were writing this book.

Figure acknowledgements

The illustrations have come from various sources and in addition to those acknowledged in the text, we also wish to acknowledge P.D. Trevor-Roper and P.V Curran's *The Eye and its Disorders* (2nd edn), P.D. Trevor-Roper's *Lecture Notes on Ophthalmology* (7th edn) and *Pocket Consultant Ophthalmology* (2nd edn), all published by Blackwell Publishing. We would also like to thank Mr Peng Khaw for the use of some of his photographs.

If we have failed to mention a specific source it is hoped that the author/publisher will accept this blanket acknowledgement and our gratitude.

Chapter 1
The Ophthalmic Patient

Introduction

The ophthalmic patient may be of any age, from a few days to over 100 years old. Ophthalmic conditions affect all age groups, though most of the ophthalmic patients seen are elderly.

Most infants and children will have parents who wish to be involved in their child's care. The child whose parents are either unable or unwilling to become involved will need the extra care and attention of a nurse to reassure him in unfamiliar and possibly frightening surroundings.

The ophthalmic patient may have other diseases such as diabetes, ankylosing spondylitis and arthritis, as these have ocular manifestations. He may also suffer from unrelated diseases. Co-morbidity can be challenging for the ophthalmic nurse who will have to make decisions about care and management based on need.

The ophthalmic patient will arrive at the eye hospital or unit either as a referral to the outpatient department or as a casualty, where many are self-referred and may not be 'emergencies' as such. They will present with a variety of conditions, from a lump on the lid to sudden visual loss or severe ocular trauma.

Most people will be anxious on a first visit to a hospital. Even for the elderly but otherwise fit person, it might be his first experience of a hospital. Those arriving following trauma will be in varying degrees of shock depending on the nature and type of accident. They and their relatives may be very anxious. Something that seems fairly minor to the nurse with ophthalmic knowledge may, to the layman, appear serious and be thought to threaten sight.

Many people have a fear of their eyes being touched, making examination difficult. Some feel faint – or do faint – while certain procedures, such as removal of a foreign body, are being performed.

There are some old wives' tales about the eye. One of the most common is that the eye can be removed from the socket for examination and treatment, and be replaced afterwards. This kind of false information does not help the patient's frame of mind.

Each person will arrive at the hospital with his own individual personality and past experience to influence any attitude towards the eye condition.

Some will be stoical, others extremely agitated. Those with chronic or recurrent eye conditions may become more used to visiting the eye hospital. Most patients having ophthalmic surgery are outpatients, day cases or overnight-stay patients. This means they have a very short time to adjust to the hospital setting and have little time to ask the questions that may be initially forgotten in the midst of all the activity. They may feel reluctant to express minor concerns when there appears to be little contact time with nurses.

The actual visual impairment experienced by the patient will vary with the eye condition. With many conditions there is no, or only slight, visual impairment and this may be temporary. Others cause gross visual loss that may have occurred suddenly or gradually over the years. This visual loss may be untreatable and permanent, may be progressive, or sight may be restored. Some patients will have only one eye affected and others both eyes, probably to different degrees. Some will have blurred vision; some will only be able to make out movements. Others will be able to differentiate only between light and dark, or will see nothing at all. Some will have lost their central vision, others their peripheral vision. Some patients will see better in bright light than dim light, and vice versa. Some degrees of visual loss can be very upsetting to the patient and prove to be a severe impairment to daily living. All patients experiencing severe visual loss will require practical and emotional help in coming to terms with it, regardless of the cause and the course it has taken.

Registration for the blind and partially sighted

Research carried out by the Royal National Institute for the Blind (RNIB) (Bruce et al., 1991) suggested that three-quarters of people eligible for registration are not in fact registered. There is no reason to suppose that this situation has changed. People are reluctant to take the final step as it can appear to be the giving up of any hope that treatment will help. But this need not be the case. Blind or partial sight registration can be a much more liberating experience for many as they realise, with help and support, that they can maximise their quality of life.

Blind register

The statutory definition for the purpose of registration as a blind person under the National Assistance Act 1948 is that the person 'is so blind as to be unable to perform any work for which eyesight is essential'. This refers to any form of employment, not only that which the patient formerly followed. It also only takes into account visual impairment, disregarding other bodily or mental infirmities. People with a visual acuity of less than 3/60 on the Snellen chart (see p. 21) or with a visual acuity of 6/60 but with a marked peripheral field defect will be eligible for registration.

Partially sighted register

There is no statutory definition of partial sight although a person who does not qualify to be registered as blind but nevertheless is substantially visually impaired can be registered as partially sighted. Those people with 3/60 to 6/60 vision and full peripheral field, those with vision up to 3/60 with moderate visual field contraction, opacities in the media, aphakia and those with 6/18 or better visual acuity but marked field loss can be included on this register. In England and Wales a Letter of Vision Impairment (LVI 2003) is obtainable from high street optometrists. In outpatient settings staff complete the Referral of Vision Impaired Patient (RVI 2003). Patients can obtain one if eligible and take this to their social services department.

Assistance and rehabilitation

The National Assistance Act 1948 directs all local authorities to compile a register of blind and partially sighted people residing in their area and to provide advice, guidance and services to enable them and their families to maintain their independence and live as full a life as possible.

Registration is voluntary. People can choose to register but if they do register they can have their names removed from the register at any time should they wish. The local authority has the responsibility of reviewing the register regularly and updating the circumstances of the people on it. Local authorities must offer services to all those identified as visually impaired, whether they choose to register or not. However, registration is necessary to qualify for financial benefits and for help from the many voluntary organisations. Registration is a good guide as to whether a person is coming to terms with their sight loss.

The process of registration starts with the ophthalmologist certifying on a form. A new system for registering as blind was introduced in England and Wales in November 2003. The Certificate of Visual Impairment (CVI 2003) replaces the old BD8. It is argued that the new system is easier to use and will speed up the process. The BP1 in Scotland and A655 in Northern Ireland are still in place that a person is eligible for either blind or partially sighted registration. The person signs this form agreeing for information on the form to be shared with their local social services, general practitioner and the Department of Population Census which maintains records of all those opting to share this information.

The Social Services Department has the responsibility of registering people. Some social services departments have delegated this task to their local voluntary organisation which deals with the blind and partially sighted people within their area. The role of the social worker is that of counsellor. They provide support and information about the services available. This includes entitlement to benefits and referral to other statutory bodies involved with retraining, special needs education for those of school and college age, rehabilitation, employment, social, leisure and recreational activities, and introduction to self-help groups.

Voluntary organisations

There are a number of voluntary organisations that work with the visually impaired. Most local areas or counties have their own organisations. These are established to provide aids and social contact for the visually impaired. Many local authorities have an arrangement with voluntary organisations to provide services to facilitate independent living such as talking or tactile watches and clocks, to alarms that sound when rained upon so that the washing can be brought in. The increase in technology has resulted in equipment being available, for example, to enlarge print onto a TV screen, to convert the written word into Braille or to use voice synthesisers.

Local voluntary organisations are often centres of social contact for the visually impaired and their carers. Some voluntary organisations maintain contact through radio stations; Glasgow for example has a radio station dedicated entirely to people with visual impairment.

The needs of people from ethnic minority groups should not be overlooked. Ethnic Enable (www.ethnicenable.com) is an organisation set up to assist people with visual impairment who are from specific ethnic groups.

Chapter 2
The Ophthalmic Nurse

Introduction

Today's ophthalmic nurse will in all probability, have been educated at university to at least diploma level. Programmes to prepare the ophthalmic nurse are offered as part of diploma, degree and masters level. Others caring for the ophthalmic patient are likely to have studied NVQ level 2 or 3 and will have gained their knowledge and skill whilst practising clinically. Within the wider workforce planning agenda other clinical roles are being developed such as assistant practitioners and surgical care practitioners.

Ophthalmic nurses will naturally be continuing to expand their practice to include for example: nurse consent; pre-operative assessment; sub-tenon's local anaesthesia; diagnosis and management of ocular emergencies (including telephone triage). The care and management of groups of patients linked to sub-specialities is not uncommon and roles include: stable glaucoma patients; oculoplastic nursing; cataract; corneal; uveitis. With any of these expanded roles, the ophthalmic nurse must be mindful of their professional accountability (Nursing and Midwifery Council, 2002).

The ophthalmic nurse must naturally possess all the qualities required of a nurse working in any speciality or environment. There are though, some characteristics that are more important to a nurse specialising in the diseases and conditions of the eye. The eye is very delicate and sensitive. Most of the patients the nurse will attend to will have varying degrees of anxiety about their eye and pain or discomfort in or around the eye. Therefore she must be extremely gentle with her hands and in her manner in order to allay any fears the patient may have about his eyes being touched. The nurse should be aware of her position and work on the patient's right-hand side when dealing with the right eye and vice versa with the left.

The eye is small and there is not much room for manoeuvre around it when performing manual nursing procedures. The nurse therefore needs to be manually dexterous. She also needs to have the best possible vision when performing nursing procedures; there is no place for vanity when dealing with the ophthalmic patient, wearing glasses for close work should these be required is essential.

As ophthalmic patients can be from any age group, the nurse needs to be familiar with the special requirements of all ages, those of the very young and the old in particular. However it is recognised that specialist paediatric nurses should as a matter of course, care for children. The difficulty here is that there are very few paediatric nurses with an ophthalmic qualification.

The nurse must be thoughtful in her approach to the visually impaired person. She must use a variety of interpersonal skills to their best advantage including: touching as appropriate to indicate presence or show concern; introducing herself; indicating when she is leaving; and never shouting. There is a great temptation to assume that a person who is visually impaired is also hard of hearing.

The nurse must always bear in mind that there is an individual human being behind the eyes that are being treated, and care for each patient as a whole, unique person.

Assessment of patients

Ophthalmic patients receive treatment as outpatients, day cases, and in primary care settings. If hospitalised, they tend to spend a minimum of time actually in hospital. Today's ophthalmic nurse has a limited amount of time in which to get to know the patient and be able to assess his needs and therefore must employ clear, succinct assessment skills in order to carry out an effective assessment. Many aspects of patient assessment may be delegated to other carers in the team. For example, a clinical support worker may measure visual acuity, take blood or record an electro cardiogram (ECG); and a technician may perform biometry.

Patient assessment remains one of the most important interactions that nurses will have with their patients and in order to do this thoroughly and efficiently requires excellent communication skills. The ophthalmic nurse must therefore, use verbal and non-verbal skills appropriately. Open-ended questions yield more information and an appropriate tone and pitch of voice should be employed. She must be aware of the effects of eye contact, facial expression, posture, gestures and touch on the patients, remembering that non-verbal communication apart from touch may not always be immediately appropriate to the visually impaired. However, if the ophthalmic nurse does not utilise her non-verbal communication skills, it could affect her own attitude and behaviour and the patient or the carer could in turn pick this up. It is also useful to integrate counselling skills such as the use of active listening, silence, and attention and paraphrasing, in order to gain additional understanding of the patient's needs. The ophthalmic nurse also needs to be very observant. The importance of clear and concise record-keeping cannot be overemphasised.

Patient information and teaching

It is well recognised by nurses that giving information about procedures for example, relieves anxiety and aids recovery. Not only do patients and carers need to know what is wrong with them and how they will be managed medically or surgically, the majority will also want to know why they are having that particular treatment. Patients and carers have ready access to Internet resources and frequently have downloaded information about their condition and treatment options. The ophthalmic nurse needs to be aware of this and be in a position to advise the patient as to the accuracy and reasonableness of this information. Many hospitals and clinics place patient information on their own Web pages as well as being available on a range of electronic media. Having an understanding of the rationale behind treatment will aid compliance and enable the patient to be actively involved. Patients and carers need information at all stages of management. Patients do benefit from effective pre-operative teaching programmes.

Today's care systems are based on multidisciplinary team-working. Nurses are not the only people who will be giving the patient information. Other health professionals such as orthoptists and optometrists also provide ophthalmic services. The role of the voluntary sector, for example HSBP (Henshaw's Society for Blind People), the IGA (International Glaucoma Association) and the RNIB (Royal National Institute for the Blind) must not be forgotten and many outpatient departments have resident representatives to assist the patient in coming to terms with their lives as people with visual impairment. Nurses are well placed to provide the patient with sufficient information about their condition and treatment. The ophthalmic nurse must, therefore, be in possession of sound knowledge in order to impart accurate information. She also needs time and the ability to use communication skills, mentioned above, appropriately. The nurse needs to assess how much information the patient needs and in what depth as well as whether to use lay or professional terminology. The ophthalmic nurse needs to be able to impart information to all age groups. As the majority of patients are elderly, she needs a special understanding of this group. Although the senses are often reduced due to the ageing process, this does not mean that the elderly cannot learn about their health needs. Visually impaired elderly people with a hearing loss are a challenge to the ophthalmic nurse, especially as loss of both of these senses may cause them some confusion.

In addition to providing information on the various conditions and their treatment, the nurse also needs to instruct the patient or carer in practical skills that need to be carried out at home, such as instilling drops, lid hygiene or inserting conformer shells. The patient or carer will need time to practise these skills following instruction from the nurse. It is vital that the nurse assesses their competence, which needs to be satisfactory if compliance is to be achieved. There are many reasons why patients fail to comply with their treatment (Williams, 1993; Patel & Speath, 1995). These include: lack of understanding of the diagnosis; if the condition is chronic; forgetfulness; lack of motivation; side effects of the drops; frequency of drop instillation; and multiple pharmacotherapy. Noncompliance may be as high as 95%, www.gpnotebook.co.uk (2003), if one takes into account late instillation or missed doses. Physical problems such as hand tremor and weakness or arthritis may be overcome by the use of devices to help in the delivery of drops.

Teaching is another area that has been affected by the shortened contact time between nurse and patient. The actual organisation of when and where to carry out teaching is often difficult. Verbal information and instruction must be backed up with the written word, both of which must be clear, unambiguous and appropriate for the individual. This includes the provision of leaflets in other languages, according to the community served. In addition, materials should be available on request in a format that the person with disability can access readily, for example Braille or tape recordings. As mentioned, many hospitals now place patient information on the Internet.

The patient's need for information and the nurse's role to give it are vitally important and, in order to save unnecessary repetition in the following text, it will be assumed under each eye condition that this is carried out.

Above all, the ophthalmic nurse needs to be a knowledgeable, competent practitioner who instils confidence in the patients with whom she has contact.

Professional issues

The ophthalmic nurse of today must be research-aware and should be encouraged to become involved in clinical research studies and clinical audit. Whilst there is an increasing body of ophthalmic nursing research, much of what ophthalmic nurses do is not research based.

Nurses are being encouraged to reflect on their practice and the ophthalmic nurse is no exception. Reflection allows time for nurses to ponder on their practice and discover ways to improve their performance. Reflection is encouraged as it goes some way to fill the theory/practice gap in nursing (Conway, 1994).

Nurses have continued to expand their roles in response to the changing demands of the service. They are increasingly undertaking roles previously carried out by doctors. Some duties previously performed by ophthalmic nurses are now within the domain of assistant practitioners and clinical support workers. They too must have the required underpinning knowledge.

Ophthalmic nurses have a key role to play in health education and health promotion. This includes informing people of how to avoid accidents in the home or work setting and screening for diseases such as open-angle glaucoma.

Ophthalmic nurses have a prime responsibility for the quality of care they deliver, regardless of the setting. The essence of care provides a useful framework for some areas of ophthalmic activity (DoH, 2003). The ophthalmic nurse can use the essence of care framework to audit her practice and to make comparisons with practices outside her own unit.

The nurse in the outpatient department

The outpatient department is the portal into the hospital or unit for the majority of patients attending with eye conditions and may be the only department they visit. The nurse working there should therefore be a good advertisement for the whole hospital or unit.

McBride (2000; 2002) has suggested that ophthalmic outpatient facilities fail to meet the needs of the patient with low vision. Nurses have a major role to play in ensuring that the environment and systems work for this category of patients and come up to a good standard.

Outpatient departments are always busy and, whilst great progress has been made in ensuring short waits for appointments (including booked appointments), there seems to be no answer to the problem of waiting time in the clinic itself. There are ways that the nurse running the clinic can alleviate the frustrations and boredom experienced due to the waiting. She can inform the patient approximately how long the wait will be and give an explanation for any delay, if possible. This may help avoid tempers becoming frayed. It is also useful to have a snack bar to direct patients and relatives to, where they can while away the time and prevent hypoglycaemia setting in – literally, in the case of diabetics. Also, advising patients about how the clinic works so they understand when for example, a patient returning from a test or investigation is not jumping the queue but rather completing their consultation.

Some outpatient departments have involved other allied health professionals in the management of some clinic cases. Optometrist lead glaucoma services is one such example. Other initiatives involve patients being seen out in primary care settings.

All patients visiting the outpatient department have their visual acuity recorded, this usually being the responsibility of the nurse. Other nursing procedures (see Chapter 3) may include:

- lacrimal sac washouts
- epilation of lashes
- taking conjunctival swabs
- removing sutures
- removing/inserting/cleaning contact lenses
- instilling drops/ointment
- removing/inserting prostheses
- testing for dry eyes using tear strips
- applying pad and bandaging
- recording blood pressure, as hypertension can be associated with retinopathies and central artery and vein occlusions; the blood pressure will need to be recorded if the patient is to undergo surgery and for general screening
- testing urine and/or blood glucose monitoring to ensure the patient is not diabetic, as diabetes can cause various ophthalmic conditions (see p. 223), and for general screening.
- minor surgery and investigations will be carried out in the outpatient department, and the nurse will need to become familiar with the procedures and instruments as she may perform the investigations herself; the following are examples of operations and tests performed under local anaesthetic:
  - incision and curettage of chalazion
  - lid surgery

- o biopsy
- o removal of lid tumours
- o retropunctal cautery
- o 3-snip operation
- o tonometry
- o perimetry
- o biometry.

The optometrist and prosthetist will normally have their clinics in this department. The prosthetist works as part of a team, with the surgeon and the oculoplastic nurse. The high number of patients attending the outpatient department poses particular problems for the nurse, as she will be unable to learn of each one's individual needs. She must be aware of those patients who require particular attention in respect of their communication and mobility difficulties. These difficulties may result from visual impairment or other physical impairments or both. These patients will usually be elderly although not always. The nurse needs to be aware of any special needs or circumstances such as diabetes, registered blind. Clinical governance dictates that confidentiality must be assured so information should be held discreetly within the notes, not pinned on the top.

The nurse is unable to see every patient as he leaves the department to ensure that he has understood any prescribed treatment or follow-up. However, she must look out for the elderly and hard of hearing in particular, in order to explain any necessary information that the doctor or practitioner may have given. This information should be supported by written information.

Some patients will have received bad news from the doctor. Those with age related macular degeneration, for example, will have hoped for treatment to improve their eyesight, only to be told that there is little that can be done apart from providing aids to assist with poor vision. Doctors need to communicate with the nurse about such patients so that the nurse is aware of these patients and available to talk to them, answer their questions and refer them to a social worker if appropriate.

The ophthalmic trained nurse will be able to give information to the patient due to be booked to come into hospital for an operation. She will be able to inform the patient of the approximate length of the waiting time for the operation, what it entails, and the length of the hospital stay. She will be able to answer any queries the patient may have. Patient assessment may be undertaken in the outpatient department at this or a subsequent visit. Pre-assessment should normally be undertaken as near to the operation date as possible to ensure that the information is as up to date as possible.

It is of benefit to the patient if he can be shown the ward or day case area. This helps allay fears of coming into hospital and is especially helpful to children and their parents.

The ophthalmic nurse working in the outpatient department has to deal with many patients in the course of a day. She needs to have sound ophthalmic knowledge to be able to attend to the wide variety of ophthalmic conditions. The eye condition may be a manifestation of a systemic disorder, so she also needs general nursing knowledge in order to give advice and to perform procedures competently. She needs to be competent in carrying out these nursing procedures and, in particular, to be aware of the special needs of the elderly, the very young, the deaf, the infirm and the anxious.

The nurse in the Accident and Emergency department

The ophthalmic nurse working in the casualty department is in a similar environment and requires the same sort of skills as the nurse working in the outpatient department. However, there has recently been a proliferation of nurse-led emergency eye services. The majority of these nurses have undertaken a recognised ophthalmic nursing qualification and have undergone a period (usually one year) of in-house training under medical and nursing supervision. These ophthalmic nurse practitioners would see any casualty patients presenting with undifferentiated ocular problems. Within the remit of their role they would diagnose, treat and refer according to protocols. In addition, the ophthalmic nurse must be able to deal with emergencies and decide on priority of care. The following conditions are considered ophthalmic emergencies and the patients will require immediate attention:

- sudden loss of vision due to:
    - central retinal artery occlusion (see p. 169)
    - central retinal vein occlusion (see p. 170)
    - giant cell arteritis (see p. 225)
    - retinal detachment – especially if the macula is still attached (see p. 165)
- primary acute glaucoma (see p. 132)
- trauma, especially penetrating or perforating injuries (see p. 203)
- chemical burns (see p. 208)
- orbital cellulitis (see p. 63).

Urgent cases the nurse may have to deal with which are not classed as emergencies include:

- corneal ulcer (see p. 106)
- vitreous haemorrhage (see p. 184)
- acute dacryocystitis (see p. 84)
- optic nerve disorders (see p. 182)
- ocular tumours (see p. 127)
- acute uveitis (see p. 123).

The nurse will need to inform the waiting patients of the approximate waiting time and she may need to explain that some people require priority care and will be attended to as soon as they arrive in the department. Locally, in response to NHS plan guidelines DoH (2000), many departments have escalation policies that 'kick in' if patient waiting times are getting too long.

It is the nurse's responsibility to take a good history and decide what priority, if any, the patient should be given. Triage is essential to ensure that real emergencies are given priority. She must give details of the state of the patient's vision on arrival and of the type of injury or eye complaint. The importance of taking an accurate history cannot be overemphasised. The history may give clues to the type of injury sustained that is not evident on initial eye examination. The history must include the following items:

- visual acuity – this may be used for medico-legal purposes especially if an accident has occurred at work and damages might be claimed
- type of injury:
  - if a foreign body entered the eye: (i) what the foreign body was; (ii) when the accident happened; (iii) how it got into the eye – it is especially important to find out whether the patient was using a hammer and chisel, and if the foreign body hit the eye with force, which might indicate that it had penetrated the eye, in which case an orbital X-ray would need to be ordered; (iv) if protective goggles were being worn at the time of the incident
  - If a fluid or powder substance has entered the eye: (i) what the substance is; (ii) when the incident occurred; (iii) whether it was washed out immediately
  - If the eye has been scratched: (i) what scratched the eye; (ii) with what force it did so; (iii) when the incident occurred
- type of eye complaint – the nurse must elicit whether the following symptoms are present and their duration:
  - discharge, especially on waking, noting the colour. In addition, age of the patient as it could be more serious in babies
  - watering
  - photophobia
  - pain or discomfort, its location and nature
  - change in vision: (i) blurred vision; (ii) floaters; (iii) visual loss (sudden; gradual; total; partial – which visual field is affected; linked to head injury?)
  - restricted ocular movement
  - any degree of exophthalmos/enophthalmos.

The patient should be allocated a triage category and treated accordingly. It should be noted that the ocular trauma could be associated with other injuries and that the latter may need to be treated before the eye injury.

If the patient has had an accident, he may need to be treated for shock. Accompanying relatives or friends may also be shocked and anxious.

Patients suffering from sudden loss of vision will be anxious, as will those who are to be admitted to hospital, especially if this is unexpected. The nurse must help alleviate these fears and anxieties. She can offer practical help such as informing relatives or arranging transport.

The nurse will be expected to carry out varied nursing procedures in the casualty department (see Chapter 3):

- the taking and recording of visual acuity
- examination of the eye – this may be carried out using a torch or with a slit lamp; ophthalmic nurse practitioners would be expected to carry out full anterior segment examination of the eye
- checking the pupils for relative afferent pupil defect (RAPD)
- instillation of drops and ointment
- removal of conjunctival and superficial corneal foreign bodies
- application of pad and bandaging
- irrigation of the eye
- epilation of lashes
- syringing of the lacrimal ducts
- removal of sutures
- removal/insertion of contact lenses
- removal/insertion of prostheses
- testing urine
- recording peripheral blood glucose
- recording blood pressure
- taking conjunctival swabs
- performing tear strip test for dry eyes
- patient education
- health and safety advice
- action to be taken if condition worsens.

The nurse must remember while performing these procedures that the patient may feel faint or unwell.

The nurse in the casualty department must be able to deal with many people and to cope with unexpected situations that might arise. She must have adequate ophthalmic knowledge to be able to recognise urgent cases and to be able to give certain patients priority care. She also needs to be able to perform a variety of ophthalmic procedures competently and knowledgeably.

This is an ideal time to carry out patient education by giving out relevant information leaflets and informing patients on eye protection as appropriate. The nurse in casualty also advises patients over the telephone so it is vital that her knowledge is accurate and her communication skills are appropriate.

The management of children with an ocular problem in an eye casualty department requires the ophthalmic nurse to be sensitive to their needs. Very young children can be frightened and anxious in unfamiliar surroundings. The parents are often equally anxious. It seems sensible to manage and treat the child quickly to ensure full co-operation during the examination process. Prolonged waiting time before children are seen will increase their fretfulness and anxiety

The day case and ward nurse

Patients in the ophthalmic day case unit or ward will require pre- and post-operative care, as the majority are admitted for surgery, e.g. cataract extraction; squint surgery; repair of retinal detachment; drainage surgery for chronic glaucoma; following trauma. There may, however, be patients admitted for rest following trauma, for intensive treatment of a severe infection, post-operative complications. The specific nursing care for each ophthalmic condition is detailed in the relevant chapters. However, a general note on nursing care is given here.

Pre-assessment

Patients having day case or inpatient surgery tend to be pre-assessed a few weeks prior to the operation. This is carried out to assess the needs of the individual patient in order to be able to plan their short period in hospital, to give the necessary information regarding the surgery and to plan with the patient and carers their care following the operation.

The care following surgery will involve instillation of drops that in the majority of cases will be performed by the patient himself or his carer. Ideally, teaching drop instillation should be instituted at pre-assessment as there is little time for this during the admission to hospital. Advising patients to purchase artificial tear drops and practise at home following instruction is one way of overcoming the lack of time there is to carry out this teaching and observation of the patient's performance.

The nurse has only limited time in which to assess the needs of the patients and must apply all her assessment skills appropriately (see p. 6).

As well as giving the usual pre-operative information to the patient, the nurse may carry out the following procedures:

* visual acuity (see p. 21)
* tonometry (see p. 51)
* biometry (see p. 53)
* ECG
* focimetry
* slit lamp examination for blepharitis.

Information leaflets regarding the surgery and hospital stay should be given to the patient to support the verbal information and instructions that the nurse will give. These can be translated into languages other than English if necessary. This, together with answering any queries the patient or carer may have, will help allay fears. Clinical governance requires that patients are actively involved in the production of patient information of any type.

Pre-operative care

In addition to the routine pre-operative care for surgery being performed under either local or general anaesthesia, the nurse may be required to carry out the following procedures, depending on the personal preferences of the ophthalmic surgeon (see Chapter 3):

- Instilling mydriatic drops prior to cataract extraction or retinal detachment surgery as the pupil needs to be dilated for such surgery to be performed
- Instilling miotic drops prior to trabeculectomy and keratoplasty
- Instilling local anaesthetic drops if the operation is to be performed under a local anaesthetic, such as G. oxybuprocaine 0.4%.

These drops are usually administered against a prescription or patient group direction (PGD).

Post-operative care

In addition to the normal post-operative care required by any patient after surgery, the ophthalmic nurse will need to follow a routine such as that described here, although this will vary to some extent according to hospital practice.

Eye care:

- Dressings – the eye will usually only be cleaned on the day following day case surgery, unless the patient is kept in hospital longer; cleaning is usually performed once a day or more frequently if indicated.
- Inspection of the eye – the eye will be examined post-operatively (see Chapter 3).
- Instillation of drops – if prescribed, given accordingly; ointment, if prescribed may be applied at night.
- Protection of the eye – eye pads or cartella shields may be worn on the first post-operative day; cartella shields are usually worn only at night for two weeks following cataract surgery.

Discharge – all patients should be given instructions about care and follow-up:

- Eye drops – patient's and carer's ability to instil drops should be checked. Ideally this will have commenced at pre-assessment. Names of drops and times of instillation must be written down.
- Cleaning the eye – if the eye is sticky in the mornings, it should be cleaned using cooled, boiled water in a clean receptacle and cotton wool or gauze. Advise patients to avoid using dry cotton wool near the eye, as fibres can get into it.
- General instructions – patients should avoid stooping down too low in case they lose their balance. If appropriate the patient should be advised to avoid anything causing increased exertion that will raise the intraocular pressure, such as lifting anything heavy. Patients should take care when they wash their hair to avoid getting soap or water into the eye as

this would cause irritation that could result in rubbing behaviour. These restrictions should be heeded for two weeks initially but are becoming increasingly less necessary with small incision surgery. They must especially take care not to knock the eye, which could cause haemorrhage or the iris to prolapse through the wound.

- Outpatient appointment – ensure that the patient has an appointment, usually for one or two weeks following discharge. Transport may need to be arranged for the day.
- Primary care – the nurse may need to arrange for a community nurse, home help, meals on wheels, for the patient prior to discharge.
- Convalescence – not used often but in some areas recuperation in a convalescent, residential or nursing home can be arranged for patients before they return to their own homes.
- Specialist procedures such as vitrectomy may require a patient to 'posture' in certain positions to ensure a satisfactory surgical outcome. To ensure that the patient complies with the posturing instructions, especially if they live alone, it may be necessary to involve other agencies such as those provided by social services and primary care.

It is helpful if all the above information and instructions are written down as well as given verbally, as there is often much detail to absorb in the excitement of going home.

Nursing procedures

The ophthalmic nurse working on the ward and in day case needs to be able to assess the patients and plan their care on an individual basis. She must understand the pre- and post-operative care required for each type of ophthalmic operation. She needs to be able to carry out certain ophthalmic procedures competently and knowledgeably. The nurse must also plan the patient's discharge in advance, ensuring that all relevant agencies are involved. She must be knowledgeable in all ophthalmic aspects in order to discuss relevant points with the patient and relatives so that the hospital stay can be made as easy and pleasant as possible for all concerned.

The nurse in the theatre

The nurse working in an ophthalmic theatre will need to be familiar with the nursing responsibilities and general duties required of any theatre nurse. In addition, she will need to know the following aspects of ophthalmic theatre nursing, though the details will vary from hospital to hospital.

Preparation of the patient

Care begins in the anaesthetic room where the nurse greets the patient and ensures their comfort on the chair or operating table. She will take a handover report from the day case or ward nurse. The anaesthetic nurse will establish that she has the correct patient, the surgical procedure for which the patient has given consent, the eye to be operated on and if marked, any relevant medical and surgical history including medications. The identity bracelet, if worn, is cross-referenced to the case notes.

Once on the operating table, the patient must be positioned safely and correctly, especially if a general anaesthetic is being administered. A Rubens pillow is used to position and support the adult patient's head and a head ring for a child. Local anaesthetic drops, if no general anaesthetic is to be given, may be instilled prior to the operation commencing.

If the patient is having the operation under a local anaesthetic, it is important that a nurse sits and holds his hand during the procedure. This not only reassures the patient but can give the nurse an indication of his condition. Intravenous sedatives, e.g. medazelam, may be given to the patient.

During the operation the patient's face will be covered with a sterile towel. This may make the patient feel claustrophobic and perhaps disorientated. Usually a supply of oxygen at 4 litres per minute with an air intake or air alone is administered to the patient. If oxygen is being given, the supply must be switched off if cautery is used, as it constitutes a fire hazard.

The nurse holding the patient's hand during local or topical procedures, in order to reassure the patient as well as to establish a communication link to pick up on patient discomfort intra-operatively, is a vital role. She will be able to feel any pressure from the patient's hand indicating that he may be feeling discomfort or pain.

The nurse will also observe the monitoring equipment, noting the pulse rate, blood pressure and oxygen saturation. Any deviation from normal will be reported to the surgeon and recorded in the nursing record.

Knowledge of the instruments

The nurse must have a good knowledge of the instruments required for each operation performed on the eye. The suture materials used in ophthalmic surgery tend to be very fine. Because of microsurgical technique some ophthalmic surgery does not require sutures.

Technique in handling the instruments

Preferably a non-touch technique is carried out, using forceps to handle the needles and sutures. The tips of the instruments should not be touched with the fingers as this may cause injury and also it may damage the instrument.

Wearing surgical gloves

Gloves with powder must not be used, as the starch it contains is an irritant to the eye. Surgical gloves containing no powder are available such as Biogel M worn by surgeons and scrub nurses for microsurgery. Latex-free gloves must be available where there is known allergy. The trend is to maximise the amount of latex-free equipment in the operating theatre.

Care of the instruments

Ophthalmic instruments tend to be small, delicate and expensive, and great care must be taken when handling them. Every piece of equipment must have its own label and each set of instruments should be labelled and numbered. Sets of instruments must not be split up. A record of which individual instruments and sets of instruments have been used for a particular procedure must be retained in the case notes. These procedures are vital to enable tracking to take place of equipment for the purposes of audit.

Instruments should be decontaminated and sterilised in specialist departments and following Department of Health guidelines. This is normally done in a central sterilisation unit. Before instruments are sent for sterilisation, the nurse should wipe micro instruments with spears dipped in water or balanced salt solution. Enzyme foam spray is used to remove detritus and protein from instruments. This procedure if followed, will help prevent the transmission of CJD. Sharps should either be disposable or retractable for safety and to prevent cross infection. Lumened instruments need to be flushed with sterile water and air according to the manufacturer's instructions. Quick rinse machines are available commercially for this purpose, delivering 120 ml H_2O and 120 ml of air.

Instruments are placed in trays lined on the base with lock down latex-free sheets which serve to hold the instruments in place securely during the wash cycle.

Sterilisation is usually by downward displacement vacuumed autoclave at a temperature of 130°C for three full minutes, the full cycle lasting 40 minutes in total. Each instrument must be seen to be in good working order, not rusted or damaged, and should be examined under a magnified light source before being sterilised.

The operation and use of equipment

The nurse must be familiar with the equipment used in the ophthalmic theatre:

- the operating microscope which is used for most intra-ocular surgery
- the cryotherapy machine used for retinal detachment surgery
- phaco emulsifier machines which are used for extracapsular cataract extractions and for vitrectomy surgery
- magnets used for removing intra-ocular and intracorneal magnetic foreign bodies; magnetic instruments are used with the magnet and must be demagnetised following use
- cautery machines:

- bipolar cautery is used on the eye and no diathermy plate is required
- macropolar cautery is used on lids and does require a diathermy plate
- laser machines
- emergency equipment such as defibrillators and suction.

The nurse working in the ophthalmic theatre must appreciate the delicate nature of the surgery being undertaken. She needs to understand the importance of quietness, speed, attentiveness, cleanliness and sterility. The nurse must also know the particular procedures for each ophthalmic operation at which she will be assisting and be prepared to develop her knowledge as new procedures and instruments are introduced.

Chapter 3
Ophthalmic Nursing Procedures

General principles

Ophthalmic nursing procedures will vary to some degree between hospitals or units. Those listed here can be used as guidelines but local policies must be followed. It is also important to remember that all ophthalmic nursing procedures should take into account patient education, infection control and health and safety.

Education of the ophthalmic patient

Most ophthalmic nursing and medical procedures carried out can seem extremely daunting to the patient and the majority of patients can be squeamish of any procedures involving their eyes. It is therefore very important that prior to any nursing and medical procedures the patient is fully informed of the nature and process of the procedure. Explanations must take into account the patient's learning style and intellectual ability, their physical and emotional state and any sensory deficits.

Infection control

Extra-ocular and intra-ocular infection can have a potentially devastating effect on the ocular diagnosis of the patient and their carers and the importance of hand washing before and after each patient contact cannot be overemphasised. Infection control also includes other measures such as employing single-use disposable items, correct decontamination and sterilisation of equipment; correct sharps and waste disposal; and observing standard and transmission based precautions.

Health and safety issues

When performing ophthalmic procedures, the patient's head should always be well supported to prevent any accidental damage to the eye. All ophthalmic procedures should be performed with a good light source and adequate magnification. Any used ophthalmic instruments should follow National Guidelines for decontamination and instructions for any 'single patient use' equipment must be stringently adhered to.

Recording visual acuity

Visual acuity is the measurement of acuteness of central vision only. An accurate assessment of visual acuity is one of the most important parts of any ophthalmic examination. Visual acuity is a test of the visual system from the occipital cortex to the cornea. Accurate visual acuity testing requires:

- patient's co-operation and comprehension of the test
- ability to recognise the forms displayed
- clear ocular media and correct focusing
- ability of the eyes to converge simultaneously
- good retinal function
- intact visual pathways and occipital cortex.

When all these criteria are present, it is a good test of macula function (North, 2001).

Common charts used in the measurement of distance visual acuity

The most common chart for measuring distance visual acuity in a literate adult is the Snellen chart.

Distance vision (Fig. 3.1)

Distance vision is tested at 6m as rays of light from this distance are nearly parallel. If the patient wears glasses constantly, vision may be recorded with

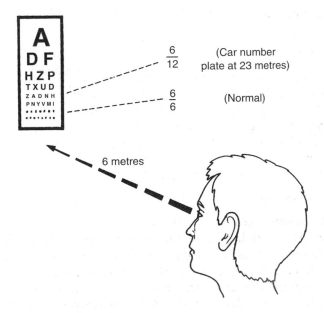

Fig. 3.1 Testing distance visual acuity.

and without glasses, but this must be noted on the record. Each eye is tested and recorded separately, the other being covered with a card held by the examiner.

Snellen's test type

Heavy block letters, numbers or symbols printed in black on a white background, are arranged on a chart in nine rows of graded size, diminishing from the top downwards. The top letter can be read by the normal eye at a distance of 60 m, and the following rows should be read at 36, 24, 18, 12, 9, 6, 5, 4 m respectively.

The patient is seated 6 m from the chart, which must be adequately lit, and asked to read down to the smallest letter he can distinguish, using one eye at a time.

Visual acuity is expressed as a fraction and abbreviated as VA. The numerator is the distance in metres at which a person can read a given line of letters. The denominator is the distance at which a person with normal average vision can read the same line, e.g. if the seventh line is read at a distance of 6 m, this is VA 6/6. If some letters in the line are read but not all, it is expressed as, for example, VA 6/6 − 2, or VA 6/9 + 2.

For vision less than 6/60 the distance between the patient and the chart is reduced a metre at a time and the vision is recorded accordingly as, for example, 5/60, 4/60, 3/60, 2/60, 1/60.

If the patient cannot read the top letter at a distance of 1 metre, the examiner's hand is held at 0.9 m, 0.6 m or 0.3 m away against a dark background and the patient is asked to count the number of fingers held up. If he answers correctly, record VA = CF (count fingers). For less vision the hand is moved in front of the eye at 0.3 m, record VA = HM (hand movement).

In the case of less vision, test for projection of light by shining a torch into the eye from different directions to see if the patient can tell from which direction it comes. If he sees the light but not the direction, it is noted as VA = PL (perception of light). This test is performed in a dark room. If no light is seen, record NO PL, which is total blindness. A 'pinhole disc' is used if the VA is less than 6/6 or 6/9, which may improve VA. If considerable increase in vision is obtained, it may usually be assumed that there is no gross abnormality, but a refractive error.

General considerations when performing visual acuity

- In order to assess accurately a patient's visual acuity (both distance and near), it is extremely important that the test type or reading material is correctly illuminated, i.e. if using a Snellen box, that all the bulbs are in working order. When testing a patient's near vision, ensure that there is an adequate light source.
- It is also important to record if a patient uses contact lenses and if these were worn at time of testing.

- Since each eye is tested separately, it is a good idea to occlude the other eye with his outpatient card or occluder to avoid patient 'cheating' by looking through the gaps between their fingers. Similarly it is a good idea to rotate the chart round for frequent attendees to the eye outpatient to minimise patients memorising the letters on the chart.
- It is important that the appropriate testing chart, such as the Sheridan Gardner test chart, Kay picture chart or the E chart (see below for explanations), is used on patients with any learning disabilities and language difficulties. Good communication skills and patience are needed in these circumstances
- The measurement of visual acuity in children also requires special skill and patience and it is important that an appropriate chart is used on those who are unable to recognise the alphabet.

Sheridan Gardner test chart

This chart can be used for children and patients who are illiterate. This test type has a single reversible letter on each line. For example, A,V,N. The child holds the card with these letters printed on. The child is asked to point to the letter on his card which corresponds to the letter on the test type. This test can be used for very young children as well as they do not have to name a letter.

Kay Picture chart

This chart is again used with patients who are illiterate or children. Instead of letters, the book contains pictures. The pictures in the book are also of varying sizes. The patient is asked what the picture represents. In order to avoid any misunderstanding amongst patients with language difficulties, it is good practice to ask the hospital's official interpreter to translate for patients.

E chart

This again is mainly used for patients who are illiterate. In the chart, the Es face in different directions. The patient is asked to hold a wooden E in his hand and to turn it the same way as the one the examiner is pointing to on the test chart.

It is important to remember that apart from the Snellen chart, any other charts used to test the patient's visual acuity *must* be written down, for example, if the Kay picture chart is used, this must be indicated in the notes.

LogMAR chart

The logMAR (Fig. 3.2) chart has been designed to overcome some of the limitations of the Snellen chart in measuring distance visual acuity. There are five letters of 'almost equal legibility' on each of the rows. Spacing

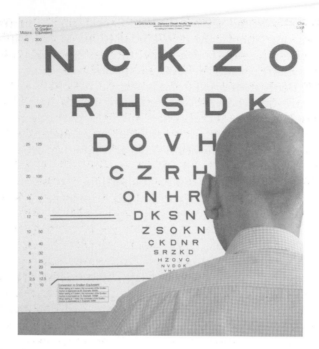

Fig. 3.2 LogMAR chart.

between letters on each row is equal to one letter width and spacing between rows is equal to the height of the letters on the smaller row. The chart is designed for a standard testing at 4 m.

Near vision

Near vision is tested by cards consisting of different sizes of ordinary printer's type, each card being numbered. The eyes are tested and recorded separately, and if the patient uses reading glasses, these should be worn during the test.

The card is held at a comfortable distance (approximately 25 cm) and should be well illuminated by a light from behind the patient's shoulder. The near vision is recorded as the card number of the smallest size type he can most easily read.

Examining the eye

Although the main focus in this section is on examining the eye, it is good nursing practice to take a holistic approach to patient care. Ensure that the patient you are going to examine is made comfortable and pain free. For any patients with a traumatic eye injury, ensure that the patient is not suffering from shock and has not sustained any other injuries. Always consider the patient's age and psychological state.

Patients attending with an acute eye problem should always have their ophthalmic history taken first to ascertain the nature and acuteness of the problem. For example, patients attending with a chemical injury treatment should always be instigated prior to examining the eye.

When examining a patient's eye, first look at the patient's face as a whole to determine facial symmetry and note any obvious palsy, ptosis, proptosis, obvious trauma, ocular movement or allergic reactions.

The eye is always examined from the outside inwards. If only one eye is affected, inspect the 'good' eye first for comparison.

Ask the patient to open both eyes as this is easier than opening one. Use a slit-lamp or a good pen torch. Ensure that the patient's head is well supported. If the patient is in pain, topical anaesthetic drops may be necessary. However, the patient's pain must be assessed before administering any topical anaesthetic. The patient's pain can be assessed using a pain-rating tool such as the verbal pain scale. Care should be taken not to 'misuse' the topical anaesthetic in controlling a patient's corneal pain since this can actually delay corneal epithelial healing. *On no account* must these drops be given to the patient to take home. If the patient is in a great deal of pain, more effective oral analgesia or a non-steroidal anti-inflammatory such as Voltarol can be prescribed.

If there is a history of glass or fibreglass in the eye or the history indicates possible penetrating injury or perforation, local anaesthetic should not be instilled. The reason for the former is to more easily identify if the glass/fibreglass has been removed; the latter to avoid the drug entering the eye.

Eyelids

Look for:

- ptosis
- swelling (see Colour Plate 1)
- discoloration
- discharge/crusting
- ingrowing lashes (see Colour Plate 2)
- entropion
- ectropion
- laceration.

Conjunctiva

The upper palpebral conjunctiva must also be examined through everting the upper lid. Look for:

- injection (redness)
- degree of injection
- position of injection:
  - limbal/ciliary
  - localised – with or without dilated episcleral vessels
  - generalised

- subconjunctival hemorrhage
- chemosis (swelling)
- foreign body (see Colour Plate 3)
- laceration
- cysts
- pinguecula
- pterygium
- follicles
- papillae (see Colour Plate 1).

Cornea

Look for:

- clarity
- corneal curvature, e.g. keratoconus
- pannus (superficial vascularisation of the cornea)
- foreign body
- abrasion
- laceration
- ulcers.

Using a slit-lamp, examine the layers of the cornea and note any abnormalities such as sub-epithelial opacities, corneal oedema, descemets folds or breaks, fresh or old keratatic precipitate or pigment on the endothelium.

Anterior chamber

Assess:

- depth (should be deep but compare with other eye)

Look for:

- hyphaema (see Colour Plate 4)
- hypopyon
- flare and cells (using slit lamp).

Iris

Assess:

- colour – compare with other eye
- clarity and pattern.

Look for:

- iridodialysis
- iris prolapse.

Pupil

Assess:

- shape (should be round – an irregular pupil could indicate synaechiae, an oval pupil could indicate acute glaucoma)
- size
- reaction
- RAPD (relative afferent pupil defect)
- position (should be central)
- colour – usually black: the red reflex may be noted (a white or grey pupil suggests the presence of a cataract; a white pupil in a baby/child indicates a cataract or retinoblastoma or pupil membranes).

Taking a conjunctival swab

Equipment

- Correct culture medium and swab stick – different ones are required for bacteria, viruses and Chlamydia.
- Appropriate request via pathology form or ward order computer.

Procedure and rationale

(1) Identify patient and check what type of swab is required. This is to ensure the correct patient receives the correct procedure and to obtain the patient's consent and co-operation.

(2) Wash hands at the beginning and end of the procedure, and at any point when your hands became contaminated. Essential in order to prevent infection from transient organisms.

(3) Assemble equipment. If both eyes are to be swabbed label swabs 'right' and 'left' in order. This is to prevent wrong swab being placed in medium.

(4) Ask the patient to look up. This is to prevent corneal damage.

(5) Swab firmly along lower fornix from nasal side outwards. When taking swab for Chlamydia more pressure is needed to obtain the organisms from the follicles, to sweep organisms away from lower punctum. It is essential to obtain as many organisms as possible.
Note: Swabs should be taken before G. Fluorescein, or a topical anaesthetic, has been instilled.

(6) Place stick in culture bottle.

(7) Wash hands to prevent cross infection.

(8) Label bottles correctly and send to laboratory.

Principles and protocol for ophthalmic medication installation/application

General principles – instilling drops

When teaching patients and carers the correct technique for cleaning and instilling drops/ointment to the eye, there are some general principles to follow (Shaw, 2001).

The aim of all eye medications is to achieve the maximum therapeutic effect from the ophthalmic medications and to minimise risks, side effects and complications associated with their use.

- The medication is delivered in a manner that avoids risk of trauma and/or cross infection. The latter includes care of drop dispenser and any drop aid used, and instillation technique.
- The drops and ointment should be administered in the correct strength, to the correct patient, into the correct eye, at the correct time and at the appropriate interval.
- All patients must have their drop technique assessed even if they are currently instilling drops for other ophthalmic conditions, e.g. chronic glaucoma.
- Maximise the opportunity for self-medication by the patient, taking into account their state of well-being. Style and technique will vary between individuals; if the patient is observed to have a drop technique that is adequate, do not change it. Where necessary, make the arrangements for district nurse support.
- In a hospital setting, a record must be kept of all drops instilled and ointment applied.
- Medication that has passed its expiry date must not be used. Any opened drops and medication must not be used after 28 days (British Medical Association & Royal Pharmaceutical Society of Great Britain, 2004).
- Patients need to know the action and the possible side effects of their medication.
- Unless directed otherwise by medical staff, ask the patient to remove their contact lenses prior to instilling drops and ointment. Depending on the patient's ocular problem, it may be necessary to advise the patient to stop wearing contact lenses until the condition has resolved and treatment is completed.
- Patients need to know that drops can sting and may leave an unpleasant taste in the mouth.
- If patients are on more than one type of drop and/or ointment to the same eye, the order of delivery should be as per pharmacy criteria.
- Normally, one drop is sufficient. Additional drops may reduce the effectiveness as this increases tear duct stimulation and outflow. It may also increase the amount of systematic absorption. In addition, any excess drops may overflow onto the cheek and over a period of time may cause skin irritation.

- The capacity of the fornix is approximately 30 μl and the average drop size is between 25–50 μl.
- With certain medications, there will be a specific request from the ophthalmologist to occlude the punctum to reduce still further any risk of systemic absorption via mucous membranes of the canaliculi, nose and mouth. However, some medications may be prescribed specifically for their action on the lacrimal apparatus and so punctal occlusion is not desirable. In addition, it is not desirable to occlude the punctum digitally following some types of surgery.
- As the period for effective therapeutic absorption of medication is from 1 to 1.5 minutes, patients should be taught to close their eyes slowly and to keep closed for a slow count to 60. Keeping the lids gently closed without squeezing reduces lacrimal duct outflow and maximises medication contact with ocular structures (Wilson & O'Mahoney, 1999).
- An appropriate time interval of approximately three minutes is necessary between each drop in order to prevent dilution and overflow.
- All medication should be delivered to the correct location. This is generally the lower fornix but can include the cornea, lids, periocular wounds and the socket.
- Drops must be stored according to manufacturers' instructions. This includes some drops to be stored in a refrigerator at all times when not in use and others only in the refrigerator before opening.
- Before using eye drops, patients – or whoever is instilling the drops – should be instructed to shake the bottle to ensure even distribution.
- Pharmacy will label all drop boxes with patient, dose, order and storage instructions. They will also have available upon request, large print labels.
- Certain medications may have an effect on vision. This effect may be transient or last the duration of the treatment.

General principles – application of eye ointment

- Ointment may be prescribed in addition to drops.
- Ointment should be applied after any prescribed drops have been instilled leaving approximately a three minute interval between medications.
- Ointment may be prescribed for structures other than the eye.
- Ointment may be prescribed for use after first dressing, and this may not happen for up to one week in the case of some oculoplastic surgery.
- If requested, visual acuity should be recorded before ointment is applied as ointment clouds vision. Any existing ointment excess is normally removed prior to taking visual acuity measurement.
- A 2.5 cm (one inch) strip of ointment should be applied to the inner edge of the lower fornix of the appropriate eye.
- The patient should close their eye and remove excess ointment with a swab.

- The patient should be advised that the ointment is likely to cause blurring of vision because of its viscous nature.
- In the case of wounds on the lids, face or eye socket, ointment should be squeezed directly onto the wound. It may be dispersed using a moistened swab. If requested to do so by the ophthalmic surgeon, the wound or scar should be massaged using the ointment.

General staff principles on eye medication

Compliance with medication or other therapeutic regimen may be defined as a 'responsible process of self care, in which the patient works to maintain his or her health in close collaboration with health care staff; instead of following rules that are prescribed, the patient shows an active commitment to self care.' (Kyngas et al., 2000).

- Drops and ointment are drugs and some eye medications will have a systemic affect other than on the eye.
- All trust/employer policies for drug administration should be followed in conjunction with these principles. This includes hand hygiene.
- Explain to the patient what you are going to do and obtain their consent and co-operation.
- Where appropriate, involve the patient/partner/carer. Involve the district nurse where it is felt necessary to ensure the eye treatment is delivered.
- Staff should be honest about effects and side effects of drops including stinging and discomfort.
- For inpatients – including any day cases – a patient already on glaucoma medication prior to surgery, should have it confirmed that any new medication prescribed is in addition to or instead of the glaucoma medication.
- Before the patient is discharged, always ensure that *all* relevant eye medications, including any that the patient may have been on prior to any ocular surgery, have been prescribed.

General patient principles on eye medication

- The medical and nursing staff will tell the patient about the drops or ointment used.
- The nursing staff will instruct the patient on when and how to instil their drops and/or apply ointment safely.
- Staff should instruct the patient about the importance of hand washing before and after instilling drops or applying ointment to help prevent infection.
- Staff must ask the patient about any current medication as this could affect the choice of treatment.
- Pharmacy and nursing staff should determine the best way to help the patient distinguish between the different types of drop bottles that have been prescribed.

- Nursing and medical staff should talk with the patient at each visit about how they are managing the drops or ointment regimen.
- Staff should advise the patient that devices are available for purchase to help with eye drop administration. These include bottle attachments to help squeeze the bottle; those to help open the cap; and those to help the patient remember to take the next drop. Information on these devices is available in the hospital pharmacy or community pharmacy. The district nurse or practice nurse may also have the relevant information.
- Remind the patient that drops and ointments are prescribed for their use only. They should be stored according to the manufacturer's instructions, which in some cases will be in the refrigerator.
- As with all drugs, advise the patient that medications should be stored in a place out of reach of children and animals.

Staff/carer procedures for drop instillation

(1) Check identity of the patient and drops/ointment against the prescription with assistant if available. Check that the drops/ointment have not expired. In order to ensure the correct patient receives the correct drops/ointment and to obtain the patient's consent and co-operation.

(2) Wash hands at the beginning and end of the procedure, and at any point when your hands became contaminated.

(3) Position hand holding bottle/dropper/tube gently on patient's forehead. This helps to prevent bottle/dropper/tube touching patient's eye if moved.

(4) Hold down lower lid with tissue/gauze square in other hand. This exposes conjunctival sac into which drop/ointment can be instilled.

(5) Ask the patient to look up. This ensures that drop falls into lower fornix and not onto the cornea which would cause patient to blink.

(6) Instil one drop into lower fornix towards outer canthus or squeeze 5 mm ointment along lower fornix from inner canthus towards outer canthus. If the drop is instilled near inner canthus it will drain straight down the tear duct before it is of any therapeutic value. Only one drop to be instilled at one time as additional drops will overflow.

(7) Release lid and ask patient to gently close eye without squeezing then count slowly to 60 before opening. This allows time for absorption of drops and helps prevent systemic absorption.

(8) Gently wipe away excess drops or ointment. This is for patient's comfort and to prevent possible drug irritation on skin.

(9) Dispose of tissue/gauze squares in nearest clinical waste bin.

(10) Sign prescription sheet, to indicate drops have been administered.

Eye care

The majority of post-operative ophthalmic patients attend for surgery as a day case and as a result may be taught to perform their own first dressing at home since some of these patients may not necessarily be reviewed the next day.

General principles

- Only clean the eye if necessary, e.g. when discharge is present.
- Staff should instruct the patient about the importance of hand washing before and after carrying out any procedure to the eye.
- Cartella shields should be washed with soap and water if necessary. The shield should be stored dry.

Inpatient – eye care

Equipment

- eye pack containing a sterile gallipot and sterile cotton wool swabs
- sachet of normal saline
- tape
- scissors.

Procedure and rationale

(1) Identify the patient, to ensure the correct patient receives treatment and to obtain the patient's consent and co-operation.
(2) Wash hands at the beginning and end of the procedure, and at any point when your hands became contaminated.
(3) Open the pack and prepare the sterile surface, so areas of potential contamination are kept to a minimum.
(4) If there is an eye pad or cartella shield, remove from patient, noting any discharge.
(5) Clean the eye with patient's eyes closed. Use one swab only, cleaning from the inside outwards.
(6) Clean along lower eyelid margin, asking the patient to look up and everting the lower lid. Use one swab only, cleaning from the inside outwards. This helps to ensure the eye is clean with no risk of contamination and protects other ocular structures.
(7) Clean along the upper lid margin by asking the patient to look down as you gently elevate the lid away from the globe. Use one swab only, cleaning from the inside outwards.
(8) Repeat if necessary. If there is stubborn discharge, lay a wet swab over the eye for a few minutes to loosen it.
(9) Inspect the eye using a pen-torch, looking for any abnormalities.
(10) Instil prescribed drops/ointment or observe patient/carer doing so to ensure patient receives correct medication appropriately.

Applying pad and bandage

Pads are now seldom applied to patients with corneal abrasions. Kirkpatrick et al. (1993) found that the corneal epithelium healing rate was significantly improved without a pad. Patients with large abrasions may find a pad, and perhaps a bandage, afford more comfort if applied firmly as the eyelid is prevented from irritating the abrasion.

If a pad is to be applied, it is important that the eye is firmly closed under the pad to avoid corneal abrasion. In some instances it is useful to apply a piece of paraffin gauze over the eyelids, then a pad or half a pad folded in two and finally a pad applied flat over the eye. This method is useful in the casualty or outpatient departments but should not be used on post-operative patients as it will put too much pressure on the globe, unless pressure needs to be applied post-operatively, e.g. to seal a leaking wound. Secure the pad with three pieces of tape. For the right eye, the first piece of tape should be placed over the centre of the pad, diagonally from 1 to 7 o'clock. For the left eye, it is placed diagonally from 11 to 5 o'clock. The second and third pieces of tape are placed each side of this central piece, parallel to it. Position the ends of each piece of tape on each other so that removal is easier and kinder to the patient. Pads may be applied to post-operative patients undergoing certain oculoplastic procedures. Cartella shields are now in common use in most ocular surgical cases instead of a pad.

In cases of chemical injury, the eye should *never* be padded.

Disadvantages of eye pads

Eye pads have several disadvantages:

- corneal abrasion can be caused if the eye is not closed under the pad
- good medium for bacterial growth
- they are flammable
- they are uncomfortable to wear
- if the lids are swollen, a lid abrasion may occur
- corneal healing rate reduced (Kirkpatrick et al., 1993).

Bandages

There are several different methods of applying an eye bandage. One method is described here which provides a secure, comfortable, effective result.

(1) Take the bandage once around the forehead.
(2) Bring it up under the ear on the affected side and over the centre of the eye pad.
(3) Repeat this twice, covering the eye pad above and below the first central turn.
(4) Take the bandage once more around the forehead and secure it.
(5) Take care when bandaging not to occlude the 'good eye' or the patient's ears.

Performing epilation of eyelashes

Ingrowing eyelashes (trichiasis) may be removed by epilation to give temporary relief from symptoms caused by their constant irritation of the cornea and conjunctiva.

Equipment

- epilation forceps
- tissues
- fluorescein minims
- slit lamp or good light magnification unit.

Procedure and rationale

(1) Identify the patient. This is to ensure the correct patient receives treatment and to obtain the patient's consent and co-operation.
(2) Wash hands at the beginning and end of the procedure, and at any point when your hands became contaminated.
(3) Sit patient with head supported to ensure safety and patient comfort.
(4) Evert lid slightly – for lower lid ask the patient to look up; for upper lid ask the patient to look down, to prevent ocular damage and for ease of performance.
(5) Remove the lash by gripping it at its root with the epilation forceps and pulling firmly in the direction of the hair growth. This is for ease of performance and to minimise discomfort for patient and to ensure the hair root is removed.
(6) Instil G. Fluorescein to see if the cornea is staining. If this occurs, a prophylactic antibiotic, e.g. Chloromycetin, may be prescribed.

The treatment must be repeated as often as required by the patient, e.g. weekly, monthly, as necessary. Patients or carers with good vision may be able to perform epilation themselves at home.

Electrolysis

Electrolysis is used to remove ingrowing lashes by means of a needle electrode applied to the lash follicle. It is a painful procedure and the lid is first anaesthetised with a local anaesthetic injection.

Cryotherapy

Cryotherapy can be used to remove lashes by applying liquid nitrogen to the offending lash follicle. This is performed by the doctor but the nurse needs to prepare the patient.

Equipment

- local anaesthetic drops, e.g. Proxymetacaine Hydrochloride 0.5% (Ophthaine)
- local anaesthetic injection, e.g. Lignocaine Hydrochloride 2%

- 2 ml syringe
- green and orange needles
- paraffin gauze
- 'shoe horn'
- lubricant (K-Y) jelly
- sterile cotton wool buds
- dressing towel
- tissues
- epilation forceps
- liquid nitrogen (cryo) container.

Procedure and rationale

(1) Identify the patient. This is to ensure the correct patient receives treatment and to obtain the patient's consent and co-operation.
(2) Wash hands at the beginning and end of the procedure, and at any point when your hands became contaminated.
(3) Lie the patient on the bed, for patient comfort and to aid procedure.
(4) Instil prescribed local anaesthetic drops to reduce discomfort.
(5) Prepare local anaesthetic injection to reduce discomfort.
(6) Insert 'shoe horn', well lubricated with jelly, into appropriate fornix. This is to protect anterior surface of eye.
(7) Cover the patient's head with dressing towel to protect area around lid being treated.
(8) Fill cryo container with liquid nitrogen in order to assist with procedure.
(9) Put cotton wool buds into liquid nitrogen and pass to doctor when ready to assist with procedure.
(10) Pass epilation forceps when required by the doctor to assist with procedure.

The patient should be warned that lid(s) may become inflamed. Cryotherapy is not used on patients with symblepharon.

Everting the upper lid

The upper lid is everted to inspect the palpebral conjunctiva over the subtarsal area. Foreign bodies, conjunctival follicles, papillae or concretions may be present.

Equipment

- cotton bud
- slit lamp or good high magnification unit.

Procedure and rationale

(1)   Tell the patient what you are going to do. Warn him that there will be a peculiar sensation. This is to obtain the patient's consent and co-operation.
(2)   Wash hands at the beginning and end of the procedure, and at any point when your hands became contaminated.
(3)   Ask the patient to look downwards to enable lid to be everted.
(4)   Take hold of the lashes of the upper lid with one hand and gently pull forwards and downwards. To enable lid to be everted.
(5)   With the other hand, place cotton bud over tarsal plate (mid lid area) Do not apply any pressure on the globe. To enable lid to be everted.
(6)   Push gently into the tarsal plate, at the same time the hand holding the lashes everts the lid. To enable lid to be everted.
(7)   Tell the patient to keep looking down to maintain eversion.
(8)   Inspect the sub-tarsal conjunctiva to examine for abnormalities.
(9)   To reposition the lid, ask the patient to look up and blink.

Removing a conjunctival or corneal foreign body

The majority of foreign bodies (such as metal) found either on the conjunctiva or especially on the cornea are usually well embedded. Removal of such foreign bodies should *never* be attempted by inexperienced staff nor without the slit lamp. Attempted removal by inexperienced staff or without the slit lamp can cause a great deal of cornea damage and may result in creating a larger cornea injury, infection and even perforation of the cornea. Using the slit lamp for removal of a corneal foreign body by experienced staff allows a thorough examination of the eye before and after removal.

Equipment

- slit lamp
- sterile green needle firmly mounted on a cotton bud
- sterile wet (minims normal saline) cotton bud
- local anaesthetic drops
- minims Fluorescein drops
- minims Lignocaine/Fluorescein drops.

Procedure and rationale

(1)   Check and record the patient's visual acuity in order to assess extent of visual disturbance and to provide a baseline measurement.
(2)   Wash hands at the beginning and end of the procedure, and at any point when your hands became contaminated.
(3)   Take and document the patient's history. The history must include presenting complaint; patient's description of his presenting signs and

symptoms; nature of injury (e.g. while grinding, hammering, chiselling); assessment of any pain or discomfort; any subjective loss of vision; the use of any appropriate eye protection at the time of injury; any previous ophthalmic problems; allergies; and any systemic and topical medications. Note any contact lens wearers. This is to accurately assess the patient prior to examination and removal of any foreign body.

(4) Examination of the anterior segment of the eye must take into account location, type of foreign body and depth of penetration. A careful search including a sub-tarsal search of the eye must be undertaken to locate any other foreign bodies or injuries to other parts of the eye. Examination techniques such as iris transillumination and Seidel test must be carried out to exclude any intra-ocular penetration. However, it is unlikely that if a corneal foreign body is located in the anterior segment of the eye, there is any ocular penetration. This is to assess and locate extent of injury.

(5) Sit patient back from slit lamp and explain your findings to him. Explain the procedure for removal of conjunctival/corneal foreign body. This is to reassure patient and to obtain the patient's consent and co-operation.

(6) Instil topical anaesthetic such as G. Tetracaine Hydrochloride (Amethocaine) or Oxybuprocaine Hydrochloride (G. Benoxinate), to anaesthetise the anterior segment of the eye prior to removal of foreign body.

(7) Bring patient back into the slit lamp and ensure that he understands the need to keep his eyes completely still during the procedure. To maintain fixation, it is a good idea to ask the patient to fixate their other eye on an object in the room. To maintain good fixation in order for the foreign body to be safely removed.

(8) Hold the patient's upper lid with your hand, to prevent patient from blinking during the procedure.

(9) Increase the magnification on the slit lamp to obtain a better view. Using the sterile green needle firmly mounted on a cotton bud, gently dislocate the foreign body. It may be necessary to gently swab the foreign body off the conjunctiva/cornea with a sterile wet cotton bud. This is to safely and effectively remove conjunctival/corneal foreign body.

(10) Continue to examine the anterior segment of the eye for signs of infiltrate. Take appropriate action if any signs noted. Note extent of injury by using a topical fluorescein.

(11) If the foreign body is metal, a rust ring may be noted. If it is difficult to remove the rust ring at that visit, patient must be instructed to come back in two days to have the rust ring removed. Meanwhile, a broad-spectrum antibiotic must be prescribed to prevent infection. The antibiotic ointment will also soften the rust and makes it easier for its removal, and help prevent infection.

(12) It is good practice to measure the patient's intra-ocular pressure as part of the examination, to detect any abnormalities in intra-ocular

measurement which may indicate other ocular damage and to assess and document baseline intra-ocular measurement.

(13) Prescribe ointment Chloramphenicol (a PGD will support the nurse practitioner to do this) four times a day for one week, to prevent infection.

(14) Accurately document all findings, including explanation of condition to patients and relatives; health education, including the need to wear appropriate eye protection; the treatment regimen; and any follow-up appointment. This may help prevent future eye injuries and should ensure patient's understanding and concordance with treatment.

Removing a corneal rust ring

Use the same technique as removing corneal foreign body. Note that when all the rust has been removed, you will observe some rust staining on the cornea. This can be safely left alone. Ensure that there is no sign of corneal infiltrate.

Taping the lower lid to relieve entropion

As a temporary measure, the lower lid can be taped to relieve an entropion. A piece of hypoallergenic tape about 1.3 to 2.5 cm ($\frac{1}{4}$ to 1 inch) in length is applied just below the lower lid margin and secured on the cheek in such a way as to bring the lower lid into its normal position. Prior to using hypoallergenic tape for this procedure, it is important to ascertain from patient that they are not allergic to hypoallergenics. When the tape is in position on the lower cheek, ask the patient to close his eyes to ensure that the lower conjunctiva is not inadvertently exposed. If the lower conjunctiva is exposed, reposition the tape.

Testing for dry eyes using tear strips

This test is performed to discern if the eyes are dry (see p. 88). It is a test of the quantity not quality of the tear film (Ragge & Easty, 1990).

Equipment

- tear test strips
- timer or watch
- local anaesthetic.

Procedure and rationale

(1) Identify the patient in order to ensure the correct patient receives the test and is prepared.

(2) Wash hands at the beginning and end of the procedure, and at any point when your hands became contaminated.

(3) Instil local anaesthetic drops if prescribed or as per PGD. This is to anaesthetise the eye for patient comfort.

(4) Prepare strips in accordance with instructions on the packet, to ensure the test is carried out correctly.

(5) Ask the patient to look up and insert the strip in accordance with the manufacturer's instructions, to ensure the test is carried out correctly. It is helpful to mark the strip R and L as appropriate, to avoid confusion between eyes.

(6) The patient may open or close his eyes during the procedure. This is to ensure patient comfort.

(7) After five minutes remove the strips and read off the result against the scale on the packet. Record the result in the patient's notes as follows:
   o right = n mm in 5 mins
   o left = n mm in 5 mins
   o if the whole strip is wet, record the result as +++.

This forms a permanent record in the patient's notes.

When performed without anaesthesia, this test measures the function of the main lacrimal gland. The irritation from the Schrimer strips stimulates the secretory activity of the main lacrimal gland. When this test is used in conjunction with a topical anaesthetic, it measures the function of the accessory lacrimal glands. Less than 5 mm in five minutes is considered abnormal.

Testing for tear film break-up time: assessing the quality of tears

The quality of tears can be measured by applying a drop of fluorescein to the lower bulbar conjunctiva and asking the patient to gently close their eyes and position the patient on the slit lamp. The patient is asked to open his eyes and to refrain from blinking. Using the blue filter of the slit lamp, the tear film is scanned and the operator starts counting from one until the appearance of the first dry spot. The time that elapses before the appearance of the first dry spot is the tear film break-up time. The normal break-up time is about 10–15 seconds. According to Vaughan et al. (1999) the break-up time is shorter in eyes with aqueous and mucin tear deficiency.

Irrigating the eye

Irrigation of the eye is performed to clean the eye thoroughly of all foreign substances, especially corrosive matter. As an emergency measure, speedy dilution of any substance is very important and irrigating the eye immediately with the nearest tap water may greatly reduce the amount of damage to the tissues.

Equipment

- pH indicator
- irrigation set
- a bottle of sterile water or sodium chloride
- local anaesthetic drops
- Desmarres lid retractor
- paper tissues
- protective plastic bibs or cape
- paper towels
- receptacle for paper towels
- receiver.

Procedure and rationale

(1) Identify the patient, to ensure the correct patient receives treatment and to obtain the patient's consent and co-operation.

(2) Wash hands at the begining and end of the procedure, and at any point when your hands become contaminated.

(3) Sit the patient in a chair with his head well supported and turned slightly to the affected side. This is to prevent irrigation fluid entering the unaffected eye.

(4) Test pH of conjunctival sac, to ascertain how long to irrigate the eye for. Post-irrigation pH should be between 7.3 and 7.7.

(5) Instil anaesthetic drops as per PGD, to anaesthetise the eye for patient comfort.

(6) Place a protective bib and paper towels around the patient's neck. This will help prevent the patient's clothing from getting wet.

(7) Place the receiver against the patient's face on the affected side. Ask the patient to hold it if no other help is available, to collect the irrigating fluid.

(8) Initially run a stream of fluid up the cheek towards the eye, to prepare the patient for fluid entering the eye.

(9) Evert the lower lid, asking the patient to look up and irrigate the lower fornix. This is to ensure all anterior surfaces of the eye, especially the fornices, are irrigated.

(10) Evert the upper lid and irrigate the upper fornix, to ensure all anterior surfaces of the eye, especially the fornices, are irrigated.

(11) Double evert the upper lid using Desmarres lid retractor if necessary. This is to ensure that no solidified material (e.g. cement) is in the upper fornix.

(12) Complete the irrigation by asking the patient to move his eye from side to side and up and down, holding the lids open. To ensure all anterior surfaces of the eye, especially the fornices, are irrigated.

(13) Re-test the pH of the conjunctival sac. Allow approximately five minutes between irrigation and pH testing as testing sooner than this would mean that you are testing the irrigation fluid still in the eye and

not the tear film. To ensure the pH is within normal limits (7.3–7.7) (Beare, 1990).
(14) Repeat irrigation until the pH is normal.
(15) Wipe patient's face dry, for patient comfort.
(16) Measure the patient's visual acuity in order to assess extent of ocular damage and to establish baseline measurement.

Notes:

- Do not hold the irrigation nozzle too close or too far away from the eye; about 2.5 cm is best. If too close it may touch the eye; if too far away the stream of fluid may not be sufficient to reach the eye.
- It may be necessary to instil local anaesthetic drops over the everted upper lid.

Syringing the lacrimal ducts

This is performed to determine whether the lacrimal drainage apparatus is blocked or patent.

Equipment
- dressing pack (if used)
- tray or trolley with:
  - 1 sterile 2 ml syringe
  - 1 disposable sterile lacrimal cannula
  - 1 sterile Nettleship dilator (punctum finder)
  - 1 ampule normal saline
- local anaesthetic drops, e.g. Pyroxymetacaine Hydrochloride 0.5% (Ophthaine)
- box of tissues
- bag for soiled tissues
- good light magnification unit
- patient's notes.

Procedure and rationale
(1) Identify the patient in order to ensure the correct patient receives treatment and to obtain the patient's consent and co-operation.
(2) Wash hands at the beginning and end of the procedure, and at any point when your hands become contaminated.
(3) Lie or sit the patient comfortably with head supported, for patient comfort and safety.
(4) Instil local anaesthetic drops over the inner canthus (as per prescription or PGD), to prevent patient discomfort.

(5)   Fill syringe with saline, attach cannula securely and ensure patency. This is for safety and to ensure equipment is not faulty.
(6)   Stand behind or beside the patient, for ease of performance.
(7)   Ask the patient to look upwards/outwards to prevent ocular damage.
(8)   With the right hand, insert the Nettleship dilator into the punctum vertically 1–2 mm. Then gently turn it horizontally towards the nose and carefully rotate it a few times between the finger and thumb to dilate the first part of the lower canaliculus. This is to ensure procedure is carried out correctly.
(9)   Remove the dilator and carefully insert the cannula following the direction of the canaliculus to a maximum of 4–5 mm, to ensure procedure is carried out correctly.
(10)   Inject the fluid slowly. Undue pressure must not be used, to prevent damage to the lacrimal structure.
(11)   Warn the patient at this stage that the saline may be felt and tasted at the back of the throat, to obtain the patient's co-operation and ensure safety.

Note:
If using disposable cannula, you do not need to use the dilator as the cannula is slim enough to be introduced through the punctum.

Result of the procedure

The result will be one of several and should be recorded in the patient's case notes:

- The saline may pass easily into the sac, through the nasolacrimal duct and trickle into the nasopharynx. The patient will taste the saline on the back of his tongue and can be told to swallow it. The result is reported as freely patent.
- There may be partial patency with some regurgitation around the cannula.
- The saline may return through the lower punctum around the cannula. This shows an obstruction near the nasal end of the lower canaliculus.
- The saline may return through the upper punctum showing an obstruction in the sac or nasolacrimal duct.
- Mucopurulent discharge may return with the saline if the sac is infected. This should be reported.

Occluding the upper punctum with a second Nettleship dilator is sometimes performed if the saline has returned via the upper punctum. Syringing is repeated to try to remove the obstruction. In this case an assistant is needed to hold the dilator in place. Syringing must not be performed by a nurse if there is an obvious swelling over the nasolacrimal sac, as infection renders the structures more prone to damage. The medical staff may use a set of lacrimal probes. These are used on infants in theatre, when the saline may be coloured with fluorescein to aid the detection of patency.

Subconjunctival injections

Small amounts of fluid (1.5–2 ml) can be injected under the bulbar conjunctiva. This form of treatment is not used as frequently as it used to be for eye infections. Here are some examples of drugs given by this method:

(1) Mydricaine no. 2 (Moorfields). This contains a cocktail of drugs, all having a mydriatic effect, in a 0.5 ml dose. It is used in uveitis to dilate the pupil when other methods have failed:
   o Atropine sulphate   1.00 mg
   o Procaine hydrochloride   6.00 mg
   o Adrenaline 216 µg.
(2) Antibiotics. These are given subconjunctivally to treat or prevent intra-ocular infection:
   o Cefuroxime   100 mg in 0.5 ml water
   o Gentamicin   10–20 mg.
(3) Steroids. Given to suppress the inflammatory process in cases of uveitis, steroids used include:
   o Betamethasone   4 mg (quick-acting)
   o Methylprednisolone   40 mg (long-acting).
(4) Local anaesthetics may be given in this manner.

Equipment

- dressing pack
- receiver with:
  o 1 ml and/or 2 ml syringe(s)
  o dark green needle
  o subconjunctival needle
  o drugs for injection
- anaesthetic drops
- gauze squares
- pad
- bandage
- tape
- sachet of normal saline
- steret
- good light
- prescribed drops or ointment (if applicable)
- prescription/case notes
- tissues.

Procedure and rationale

(1) Identify the patient. Explain the procedure. In order to ensure the correct patient receives treatment and to obtain the patient's consent and co-operation. It will also reduce anxiety.

(2)   Wash hands at the beginning and end of the procedure, and at any point when your hands become contaminated.
(3)   Give prescribed analgesia (if necessary), to reduce patient discomfort.
(4)   Position the patient lying down or sitting in a chair with the head well supported, to ensure patient comfort and safety.
(5)   Commence instilling local anaesthetic drops as per prescription or PGD, e.g. G. Amethocaine Hydrochloride 2% or G. Cocaine Hydrochloride 5%, one drop every five minutes over 25 minutes. To reduce patient discomfort, cover eye with cartella shield, to prevent damage to the cornea.
(6)   Prepare drugs to be injected. Check with second nurse to ensure safety. Put subconjunctival needle on syringe firmly and check potency.
(7)   Once eye is anaesthetised commence procedure.
(8)   Open dressing pack as usual.
(9)   Clean eye if necessary.
(10)   Hold lower lid down and ask patient to look up (an assistant may be required). To ensure procedure is carried out correctly.
(11)   Hold the syringe horizontally, the needle bevel uppermost and fingers in the correct position to inject the drug, to ensure procedure is carried out correctly.
(12)   Insert the needle under the conjunctiva in the folds of the lower fornix.
(13)   Inject the drug slowly. The conjunctiva will balloon forwards as it is injected.
(14)   On completion of the injection withdraw needle.
(15)   Insert antibiotic ointment or drops if prescribed, to prevent infection.
(16)   Apply pad and bandage for four hours, for patient comfort.

Notes:

- Methylprednisolone must not be mixed with any other drug.
- If no assistance is available, it may be necessary to use:
  ○ a speculum to hold the lids open
  ○ Moorfields forceps to hold up the conjunctiva to ease the insertion of the needle.
- Analgesics may be given before the procedure and again once the local anaesthetic has worn off.

Inserting/removing a contact lens

Procedure and rationale

Insertion of a contact lens

(1)   Wash hands at the beginning and end of the procedure, and at any point when your hands become contaminated.
(2)   Place contact lens on tip of index finger, to aid insertion.

(3)   Hold the lids apart with the other hand and ask the patient to look straight ahead. To prevent lids blinking during insertion and to position eye correctly.
(4)   Place the lens over the cornea. To correctly position the lens.
(5)   Ask the patient to blink in order to centre lens in correct position.
(6)   If an extended wear or bandage lens is being inserted, because they are larger, it may be necessary to evert the lower lid first and place the lens in the lower fornix. Then ask the patient to look down while you place the upper lid over the top of the lens.

Removal of a contact lens

If possible ask the patient to remove his lens himself. This is always easier, as people develop their own particular method. If you have to do it:

(1)   Wash hands at the beginning and end of the procedure, and at any point when they become contaminated.
(2)   For hard or gas permeable lenses: place your index finger on the lens and gently move it to one side of the cornea and pull away. The eyelids can be used to lever the edge of the lens away from the cornea. A small rubber suction extractor can be used. This is squeezed between the thumb and index finger and placed on the lens. The pressure of the thumb and finger is released and the suction thus caused removes the lens with the extractor as the latter is pulled away from the eye. For soft, extended wear and bandage lenses: gently squeeze the lens between thumb and finger and remove it. Place in correctly labelled container, with normal saline solution.

Inserting/removing a prosthesis/shell

Inserting a prosthesis/shell

(1)   Tell the patient what you are going to do.
(2)   Wash hands at the begining and end of the procedure, and at any point when your hands become contaminated.
(3)   Pull up the upper lid and insert the prosthesis into the upper fornix.
(4)   Evert the lower lid and slip lower border of the prosthesis into the lower fornix.

Removing a prosthesis/shell

(1)   Tell the patient what you are going to do.
(2)   Wash hands at the begining and end of the procedure, and at any point when your hands become contaminated.
(3)   Evert the lower lid and ease the prosthesis out. A small plastic spatula may be required to assist in the removal. The prosthesis then slips out.

Removing a dacryocystorhinostomy tube

Equipment

- nasal speculum
- stitch scissors
- long Spencer Wells forceps
- torch.

Procedure and rationale

(1) Identify the patient to ensure the correct patient receives treatment and to gain the patient's consent and co-operation.
(2) Wash hands at the beginning and end of the procedure, and at any point which your hands become contaminated.
(3) Ask the patient to blow his nose, especially down the nostril on the affected side to enable the tube to be more easily removed.
(4) Position patient in chair, for comfort and safety.
(5) Clasp the tube in the nostril with forceps to ensure procedure is carried out correctly.
(6) Cut the tube in the inner canthus to ensure procedure is carried out correctly.
(7) Pull the tube out from the nostril.

Note:
The snip and blow method used by the ophthalmologist for removal of a dacryocystorhinostomy tube involves instilling topical anaesthetic in the operated eye. Lignocaine spray is sprayed into the nostril and the patient is told to blow his nose. An endoscope is inserted into the nostril and the tube is snipped from the upper and lower punctum. The tube is gently pulled from the nostril using a curved forcep. Occasionally, if there is a lot of mucus which is adherent to the tube, gentle suction can be applied up the nostril prior to removal of the tube.

Preparing a patient for fundal fluorescein angiography

Procedure

(1) Check that all relevant documentation, i.e request form for fluorescein angiogram has been signed.
(2) Check patient's details, e.g date of birth and address correspond to fluorescein request form.
(3) Explain procedure to the patient:
    o dilating drops will be instilled in the eye/eyes to be photographed
    o initially colour photographs will be taken followed by black and white photographs
    o a fluorescein dye will be injected into the ante-cubital fossa or dorsal aspect of the hand via a butterfly or Venflon

- o the dye normally takes about 6–10 seconds before appearing at the fundus
- o patient will be asked to look at a fixation point during the procedure
- o patient will be warned about their skin discolouration and the urine being discoloured for 4–6 hours
- o patients are also informed about the side-effects of fluorescein – ranging from mild nausea, vomiting, urticaria, rash, bronchospasm and anaphylactic shock.

(4)   Obtain the patient's medical history, medications and allergies.

(5)   Obtain written consent from patient.

Notes:

- Proceed with caution in patients with severe allergies to other dyes or medicines, severe asthmatics and very recent cardiac problems.
- Pregnant women should never be given IV (intravenous) fluorescein.
- Breast-feeding women should be warned that the fluorescein dye will be exhibited in their breast milk and therefore should not breast-feed their baby for 24 hours.
- All relevant emergency drugs and equipment must be at hand for any potential complication.
- Extravasation must be avoided as it is extremely painful for the patient.
- Patients who frequently experience nausea or vomiting can be prescribed oral Buccastem, an anti-emetic ½ hour before the procedure. One to two tablets are placed high between upper lip and gum and left to dissolve. Record all reactions to IV fluorescein in the patient's notes
- Before dilating any ophthalmic patients, check the type of intra-ocular lens in situ (iris clips cannot be dilated). Contact lenses should normally be removed unless specifically instructed not to by the doctor.

Preparing a patient for intravenous injection of indocyanine green dye

Indocyanine green (ICG) has been used for more than 30 years in tests of cardiac and hepatic functions (Lund-Johansen, 1990). The use of ICG in ophthalmology to study the circulation of the retina – and especially of the choroid – is of particular value. Indocyanine green angiography, like fluorescein, is generally considered to be a safe procedure but being invasive, adverse reactions very similar to fluorescein are known to occur. Reactions range from mild nausea and vomiting, sneezing, urticaria, syncope to severe reactions affecting the cardiac and respiratory systems.

Any patient requiring a ICG angiography should be screened for allergic reactions especially to iodine, shellfish or previous reaction to ICG. ICG has a 'thinner' feel than fluorescein and enters the body much more quickly than fluorescein.

The recommended dose for ICG is 25 mg in 5 ml of aqueous solvent. A 5 ml bolus of normal saline should immediately follow the injection.

Radioactive iodine uptake studies should not be carried out for one week following ICG angiography.

Since ICG is removed from the bloodstream exclusively by the liver, the dye will ultimately be excreted with intestinal contents, so no skin discolouration will occur.

Notes:

- Resuscitation equipment must be at hand as Fluorescein and Indocyanine green can cause anaphylactic shock.
- The patient must stay for half an hour following the angiogram to enable observation for any reaction to the dye.

Preparing a patient for laser treatment

Procedure

(1) Take visual acuity.
(2) Wash hands at the beginning and end of the procedure, and at any point when your hands become contaminated.
(3) Explain the procedure to the patient:
   o mydriatics will be instilled if the retina is to be treated and maybe for a capsulotomy
   o local anaesthetic drops will be instilled
   o the patient will have to keep his eyes very still while flashing green lights are emitted from the argon laser; usually nothing is noted by the patient receiving laser treatment from the YAG laser
   o following capsulotomy and trabeculoplasty, the intraocular pressure will be measured one hour after the procedure.
(4) Wipe eyes following the procedure. Lubricating jelly will have been used for the contact lens.

Notes:

- Staff in the laser room should wear protective spectacles and adhere to laser safety policies.
- In order to prevent a hypoglycaemic/hyperglycaemic attack during laser treatment, ensure that patient has had their required intake of food and relevant anti-hypoglycaemic agents.
- Inform patient of alternative analgesia such as entonox or peribulbar injection.
- Whilst it is important for patient to keep still during laser treatment, inform the patient of alternative means of communicating with the doctor during treatment such as tapping on the laser table to gain the doctor's attention.
- For indirect argon laser, the patient will have to be laid down.

Preparing a patient for photodynamic therapy (PDT)

Procedure

(1) Full explanation must be given to the patient.
(2) The patient's visual acuity is measured using the logMAR.
(3) Wash hands at the beginning and end of the procedure, and at any point when your hands become contaminated.
(4) The patient blood pressure, pulse rate, height and weight are all accurately measured and recorded. The patient's height and weight is necessary to calculate the dosage of the Visudyne (Verteporfin).
(5) An identification bracelet is attached to the patient's wrist and it is essential that correct details are recorded and the patient wears the band for at least 48 hours following treatment to remind the patients as well as other health professionals that they have received Visudyne therapy.
(6) The patient pupil is dilated.
(7) The Visudyne infusion equipment is prepared and set up.
(8) The Visudyne is given via a cannula.
(9) Post treatment information included avoiding sunlight for 48 hours, wearing of sunglasses and to wear clothing that will fully cover their arms and legs. Patients should be warned that their vision might be blurred. Other adverse reactions to the Visudyne therapy including back pain during infusion, severe decreasing vision and reactions around the cannula site such as pain, swelling, hypersensitivity and leaking of Visudyne around cannula site.

Preparing a patient for ultrasound

Procedure

(1) Take visual acuity.
(2) Explain the procedure to the patient:
   o   local anaesthetic drops will be instilled
   o   dilating drops will be instilled
   o   keratometry will be performed prior to an A-scan
   o   the patient will need to look ahead and keep his eyes still while the scan is being performed.

Applying heat to the eye

Heat can be applied to the eye in several ways to reduce swelling, encourage the discharge of infected cysts, ease pain and enhance the action of drugs – especially mydriatics. Patients must be assessed as to their ability to safely comply with the procedure.

Application of heat using a clean flannel

A clean flannel is put under a hot tap (as hot as the patient's hand can stand). It is wrung out and applied to the closed eyelid. As the flannel cools down, this procedure is repeated a few more times.

Thermos flask

A thermos flask is filled with hot water. The head is positioned so that the steam rising from the flask bathes the closed eye.

The danger of scalding from both methods must be remembered.

Removal of sutures

Equipment

- sterile receiver with fine scissors; stitch cutter; or blade
- 1 pair fine forceps
- sachet of sterile normal saline
- gallipot
- dental rolls, cotton wool balls or gauze squares
- patient's notes.

Procedure and rationale

(1) Identify the patient and the site of sutures with doctor's instructions for removal, in order to ensure the correct patient receives treatment at the correct site and to obtain the patient's consent and co-operation.

(2) Sit the patient with his head supported and in a good light, for safety and ease of performance.

(3) Wash hands and prepare the equipment.

(4) If necessary, check with the doctor prior to the procedure, to ensure healing has occurred.

(5) Clean the suture line if necessary.

(6) Remove the sutures in order to complete the procedure.

(7) Check the suture line to ensure it is clean and intact/healed.

(8) Clear away the equipment and wash hands, in order to prevent cross infection.

(9) Instruct the patient on any follow-up advice, for continued care of the patient.

(10) Record in the case notes the fact that the sutures have been removed, as a permanent record of procedure having taken place.

Preparing the patient and equipment for minor surgery

Equipment

Trolley with:

- relevant sterile instrument set
- extra instruments
- one sheet sterile wax paper
- two sterile linen towels or paper towels
- eye pad
- several dental rolls
- several gauze swabs
- local anaesthetic drops
- local anaesthetic injection
- syringes and needles
- Mediprep or similar skin preparation
- sutures
- specimen pot with formaldehyde and pathology form if necessary
- surgical gloves
- tape.

Procedure

(1)   Identify patient and check notes about the procedure to be performed.
(2)   Wash hands then clean and lay trolley as required.
(3)   Lie the patient on couch ensuring comfort.
(4)   Ensure that there is a good light source.
(5)   Instil local anaesthetic drops prescribed by doctor.
(6)   Prepare local anaesthetic injection.
(7)   Clean around the eye with Mediprep or similar preparation.
(8)   Assist the doctor during the procedure.
(9)   Apply ointment/pad/bandage at the end of the procedure if necessary, which may need to be renewed before the patient goes home.
(10)   Explain any follow-up procedure and offer tea and biscuits.
(11)   Clear away the trolley and wipe the instruments before sending them for sterilization.
(12)   Complete minor operations register.

Note:
In some ophthalmic hospitals and units, ophthalmic nurses are performing minor operations such as incision and curettage of chalazion.

Goldmann applanation tonometry

Goldmann applanation tonometry measures the intra-ocular pressure indirectly by measuring the force necessary to flatten a 3.06 mm diameter portion of the corneal surface. The higher the intra-ocular pressure, the greater the force required.

Measuring principle (devised by Imbert-Fick)

The cornea is flattened with a plastic prism which has a flat anterior surface and a diameter of 7.0 mm. The prism is brought into contact with the cornea by advancing the slit lamp. The measuring drum, which regulates the force applied to the pressure arm, is turned and the tension on the eyes is increased until a surface of known and constant size of 3.06 mm is flattened. The intra-ocular pressure (in mmHg) is found by multiplying the drum reading by ten.

Procedure and rationale

(1) Ensure that the slit lamp is switched on and that the eye pieces are correctly focused. This ensures accurate reading of intra-ocular pressure.
(2) Switch on the blue filter and bring into the beam of the slit lamp.
(3) Adjust the angle between the illumination and the microscope to about 60°.
(4) Insert the tonometer into the slit lamp base plate. The instrument can be used in either of two positions; observation is monocular with either the right or left microscope.
(5) Bring the pressure arm into the notch position so that the axis of the prism and the microscope coincide.

Preparing the patient

(1) Identify the patient in order to ensure the correct patient receives the treatment and to obtain the patient's consent and co-operation.
(2) Check if the patient is wearing contact lenses, if so then remove them before commencing the procedure. It is not possible to perform tonometry with contact lenses in situ.
(3) Wash hands and instill topical anaesthesia into both eyes in order to reduce discomfort.
(4) Instill Fluorescein stain by means of fluorescein paper strips or fluorescein drops. For accurate reading and to prevent too much fluorescein in the eye.
(5) Instruct the patient to look straight ahead with both eyes wide open. If necessary, the patient's eyelids should be held apart by the examiner without pressure being applied to the eyeball.

For accurate measurement

Measurement:

(1) The prism is brought into contact with the centre of the cornea, by advancing the slit lamp. A blue light illuminates the limbus when

contact is made. The examiner looks through the microscope at this point.

(2) Upon contact, a thin circular outline of Fluorescein is produced. The prism splits the circle into two semi-circles coloured green. Any necessary adjustment is made by the control lever or height adjustment control on the slit lamp, until the flattened area is seen as two semi-circles of equal size in the middle of the field of view.

(3) The pressure on the eye is increased by manually adjusting the measuring drum on the tonometer, until the inner borders of the two fluorescein rings just touch each other open. The inner border of the ring represents the demarcation between the cornea flattened by applanation and the cornea not flattened.

(4) The amount of force required to do this is translated by the scale into a pressure reading of mmHg, which is found by multiplying the drum reading by ten.

Tonometry can also be performed using the handheld Perkins' tonometer or a tonopen.

Notes:

- It is good practice to calibrate the tonometer daily. Any errors in reading should be reported and documented.
- The use of disposable tonoshield or tonosafe is encouraged to prevent the spread of infection.

Keratometry

Keratometry is used to measure the greater and lesser curvatures of the cornea, usually in conjunction with biometry, to discover the strength of the intra-ocular lens required by a patient following cataract extraction. As biometry involves contact with the eye that may distort it slightly, keratometry should be performed before biometry. Each eye is tested separately. There are a number of machines used but the principles of each are similar. The patient should be sat comfortably with his chin and forehead on the rests and asked to look down the barrel of the keratometer. The patient must keep as still as possible. The nurse looks through the eyepieces and may need to adjust the machine until she sees the cornea clearly and certain points that must be aligned before a reading can be taken.

Biometry

This uses an A-scan to measure the axial length of the eye. As a probe touches the eye, a local anaesthetic must be instilled in the patient's eye. The patient is positioned comfortably with his chin supported on a rest such as a slit lamp and asked to fix his gaze. The nurse must also ensure that she is comfortable and within easy reach of the footplate. Once the patient's eye is aligned, the nurse gently places the probe on the cornea. A steady hand is required, as the probe must make contact to measure correctly. Excess pressure however will indent the cornea and give a false reading which the nurse must be able to identify.

By measuring both eyes a comparison can be made to further prove accuracy, as it is unusual to find a marked difference between the axial lengths of the two eyes. It may be easier to obtain a reading after the pupil has been dilated. The information gained from the keratometry and biometry is fed into a computer, which produces the desired intra-ocular lens power for the individual patient.

Perimetry

This is performed to assess the degree of peripheral and central visual loss. Again there are different machines in use but the principles are similar. The patient must be made comfortable as the procedure can take a long time. The patient is asked to position his chin and forehead on the rests and to fixate on a target. One eye is tested at a time, the other eye being covered. The patient indicates that he can see various lights being presented to him either verbally or by pressing a buzzer. Most machines are computerised, the result appearing on a printout. The majority of patients having perimetry are elderly and need to be encouraged to perform the task as their concentration may not be very good.

Chapter 4
The Globe: a brief overview

Introduction

This chapter is deliberately brief to avoid repetition, as more detailed descriptions can be found in the individual chapters on each structure. Its aim is to enable you to see the interrelations of the various structures.

The globe or eyeball is situated in the bony socket or orbit (see p. 59), which affords it protection. Also in the socket are nerves, muscles, blood vessels and fat.

Anteriorly, the globe is also protected by the upper and lower eyelids (see p. 60), which contain muscles, secretory glands and eyelashes.

The lacrimal gland (see p. 79) sits in the upper outer aspect of the frontal bone of the orbit and produces tears. These tears drain into the lacrimal drainage system (see p. 80). This is composed of an upper and lower punctum situated on the inner aspects of the upper and lower lid margins, the upper and lower canaliculi and the lacrimal sac, which opens into the nasal duct.

There are six extra-ocular muscles (see p. 186), which move the eye in the direction of gaze. There are four recti muscles and two oblique muscles.

The conjunctiva lines the lids (the palpebral conjunctiva) and overlies the sclera (the bulbar conjunctiva), terminating at the cornea.

The globe (fig. 4.1) is approximately 2.5 cm in diameter by the age of three years. It has three layers:

(1) The outer protective layer comprises the sclera (see p. 105) for approximately its posterior five-sixths and the cornea (see p. 103) for its anterior one-sixth. The cornea is clear to allow light rays through and is highly sensitive. The sclera is composed of tough white fibrous tissue.

(2) The middle layer is the pigmented vascular uveal tract (see Chapter 9). The choroid forms approximately the posterior four-fifths and the ciliary body and iris the anterior one-fifth. The iris is a diaphragm allowing varying amounts of light to enter the eye through the pupil in its centre. The ciliary processes produce aqueous and the ciliary muscles control the shape of the lens for focusing. The choroidal blood vessels supply the underlying outer layers of the retina.

(3) The inner layer is formed by the retina (see p. 160) and is the nerve ending layer containing rods and cones, which receive the light

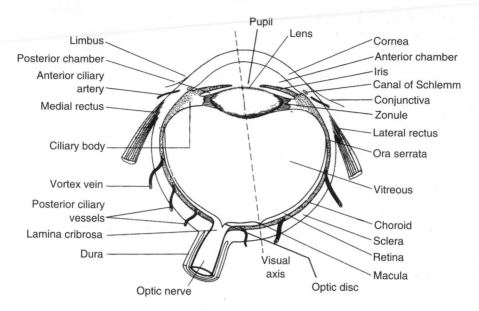

Fig. 4.1 Diagrammatic horizontal section of the eye.

stimulus that is sent via the optic nerve to the occipital cortex for interpretation.

Aqueous (see p. 130) is produced by the ciliary processes, which are part of the ciliary body, and flows into the posterior chamber, through the pupil, into the anterior chamber and drains through the trabecular meshwork and the canal of Schlemm in the angle of the anterior chamber. There is also some drainage via the uveo-scleral route. It nourishes the lens and cornea.

The anterior chamber (see p. 130) is the area between the cornea and the iris.

The posterior chamber (see p. 130) is the area between the posterior surface of the iris and the anterior surface of the lens.

The crystalline lens (see p. 148) is suspended by the suspensory ligaments (zonules) from the ciliary body and lies behind the iris. It is clear to allow light rays to pass through unhindered. It changes shape so light rays can be focused on the retina for near vision, a process known as accommodation.

Vitreous (see p. 164) is a clear gelatinous substance, which fills the posterior segment of the eye between the lens and the retina.

The nerve supply to the eye

The oculomotor or third cranial nerve supplies the:

- levator palpebral superioris muscle
- superior rectus muscle

- inferior rectus muscle
- medial rectus muscle
- inferior oblique muscle.

Its branch, the short ciliary nerve supplies the:

- sphincter muscle of the iris
- ciliary muscle.

The trochlea or fourth cranial nerve supplies the:

- superior oblique muscle.

The trigeminal or fifth cranial nerve. The first division of the trigeminal nerve is the ophthalmic division. This division has three branches:

- lacrimal, supplying the lacrimal gland
- frontal, supplying the skin of the forehead
- nasociliary, with two branches:
  - infratrochlea supplying the inside of the nose
  - long ciliary supplying the dilator muscle of the iris, the conjunctiva and the cornea.

The abducens or sixth cranial nerve supplies the:

- lateral rectus muscle.

The facial or seventh cranial nerve supplies the:

- orbicularis muscle.

The blood supply to the eye

The ophthalmic artery and its branches supply the blood to the eye. Drainage is via the ophthalmic vein and its branches:

- The central retinal artery and vein supply and drain the retina.
- The short posterior ciliary artery and choroidal vein supply and drain the choroid.
- The long posterior ciliary artery supplies the ciliary body.
- The anterior ciliary artery supplies the:
  - ciliary body
  - conjunctiva
  - corneal limbus.
- The arterial circle of the iris, supplying blood to the iris, is formed from the:
  - long posterior ciliary artery
  - anterior ciliary artery.

- The anterior ciliary vein drains the:
  - ciliary body
  - iris
  - conjunctiva
  - corneal limbus.
- The conjunctival artery and vein supply and drain the conjunctiva.
- The superior and inferior medial palpebral artery and vein supply and drain the:
  - conjunctiva
  - eyelids
  - lacrimal sac.
- The episcleral artery and vein supply and drain the sclera.
- The lacrimal artery and vein supply and drain the:
  - lacrimal gland
  - eyelids.
- The supra-orbital artery and vein supply and drain the upper eyelids.
- The muscular artery and vein supply and drain the extra-ocular muscles.
- The nasal artery and vein supply and drain the lacrimal sac.
- The frontal artery and vein supply and drain the forehead.
- The four vortex veins drain the ciliary body, iris and choroid leaving the globe at its equator to drain into the ophthalmic vein.

Chapter 5
The Protective Structures

The orbit

The eyeball or globe is protected by the bony socket or orbit in which it sits (Fig. 5.1). The orbit is composed of seven bones:

- maxilla
- frontal
- lacrimal
- ethmoid
- sphenoid
- zygomatic
- palatine.

Each orbit has four walls: a floor, roof, lateral wall and medial wall. The two medial walls are parallel to each other and the two orbits diverge to allow for a greater field of vision. The orbits are pyramid-shaped with the apex posteriorly.

Areas of the orbit

- Roof: triangular-shaped and made up of the frontal bone anteriorly and part of the sphenoid posteriorly.
- Floor: triangular-shaped and made up of the maxilla anteriorly, part of the zygomatic laterally and the palatine posteriorly.
- Lateral wall: composed of the zygomatic anteriorly and the sphenoid posteriorly.
- Medial wall: composed of four bones; from the front backwards: part of the maxilla, the lacrimal, the ethmoid and part of the sphenoid.

Three apertures are situated at the apex of each orbit:

(1) The optic foramen through which passes:
  - the optic nerve (second cranial nerve) leaving the orbit (see optic pathways, p. 163)
  - the ophthalmic artery entering the orbit, running underneath the optic nerve.

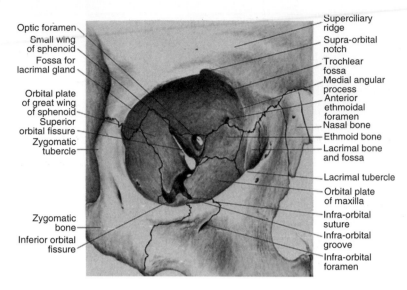

Fig. 5.1 The orbit from in front.

(2)   The superior orbital fissure through which pass:
  (a)   nerves:
      (i)   oculomotor (third cranial nerve) – superior and inferior branches
      (ii)   trochlea (fourth cranial nerve)
      (iii) trigeminal (fifth cranial nerve) – three branches of the first division (ophthalmic division): lacrimal, frontal and nasociliary
      (iv)   abducens (sixth cranial nerve)
  (b)   blood vessels:
      (i)   ophthalmic vein – superior and inferior branches.
(3)   The inferior orbital fissure through which pass:
  (a)   the infra-orbital artery
  (b)   the trigeminal nerve – some branches of the second division (maxillary division).

Surrounding the globe in the socket are muscles, ligaments, blood vessels, nerves and fat. Tenons capsule is a thin membrane which encircles the globe from the margin of the cornea to the optic nerve, adhering closely to the sclera beneath it.

The eyelids

The functions of the eyelids are to protect the globe and to lubricate its anterior surface (Fig. 5.2). The top lid, the larger of the two, closes over the globe to protect it. By blinking, the tear film is spread over the anterior surface thus lubricating it (see p. 82).

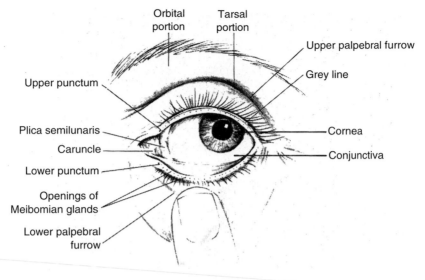

Fig. 5.2 The outer appearance of the eye and eyelid.

Areas of the lid

These are illustrated in Fig. 5.3:

- Palpebral conjunctiva lining the under-surface.
- Tarsal plate – a band of connective tissue lying posteriorly forming a stiff plate.
- Skin on the outer surface.
- Grey line – inter-marginal sulcus, where the skin joins the palpebral conjunctiva on the lid margin.
- Hair follicles – lashes, near the grey line.
- Fat – surrounding the structures.
- Glands:
  - Meibomian glands. There are 20–30 Meibomian glands in each lid, contained within the tarsal plate, their ducts opening through the palpebral conjunctiva just behind the lashes. They produce a sebaceous substance which creates the oily layer of the tear film (see p. 81).
  - Glands of Moll: these are sweat glands producing sebum.
  - Glands of Zeis: these are modified sebaceous glands which open into the lash follicles.
  - Glands of Krause and Wolfring: these are situated in the fornices and are accessory tear glands.
  - Sweat glands: these open directly onto the skin of the outer surface.
- Muscles – there are three muscles supplying the eyelid:
  - orbicularis:

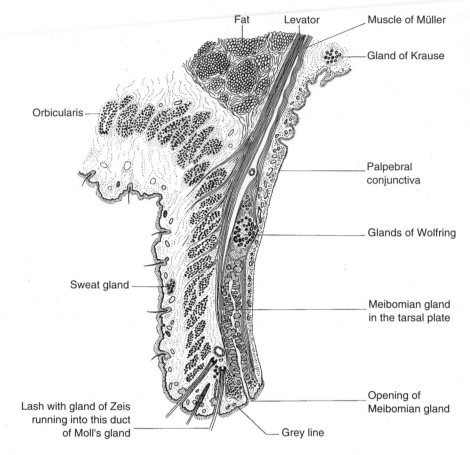

Fig. 5.3 Vertical section through the upper lid.

      (i)   origin – lacrimal bone
      (ii)   insertion – deep in the fascia around the lacrimal sac
      (iii)   function – to close the lids and to screw up the eyes
      (iv)   nerve supply – facial nerve (seventh cranial nerve)
o   levator palpebral superioris:
      (i)   origin – Annulus of Zinn (a ring tendon surrounding the optic nerve at the apex of the orbit)
      (ii)   insertion – into the tarsal plate, palpebral ligaments and skin of the upper lid
      (iii)   function – to lift the upper lid
      (iv)   nerve supply – oculomotor (third cranial nerve)
o   Müller's muscle (this is a smooth muscle):
      (i)   origin – in the levator palpebral superioris muscle
      (ii)   insertion – tarsal plate
      (iii)   function – to provide extra elevation to the upper lid
      (iv)   nerve supply – sympathetic nervous system.

Sensory nerve supply

Upper lid: ophthalmic division of the trigeminal nerve (fifth cranial nerve).
Lower lid: maxillary division of the trigeminal nerve.

Blood supply

The blood supply to and drainage from the eyelids is via:

- lacrimal artery and vein
- supra-orbital artery and vein (upper lid)
- superior and inferior medial palpebral artery and vein.

Conditions of the orbit

Orbital cellulitis

Orbital cellulitis (Fig. 5.4 and Colour Plate 5) is an acute purulent inflammation of the cellular tissue of the orbit. It is an ophthalmic emergency because of optic nerve compression. It is more common in children and is usually unilateral.

Causes

- Spread of infection from neighbouring structures, e.g. nasal sinus.
- Sepsis following penetrating injuries.
- Following septic operations, e.g. enucleation.
- Facial erysipelas.
- Spread of pyaemia – causative organisms: *Pneumococcus*; *Staphylococcus*; *Streptococcus*.

Signs

- Proptosis of the affected eye, pushed forward by the inflamed tissue within the orbit, behind the eyeball.

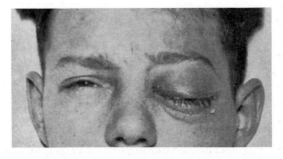

Fig. 5.4 Orbital cellulitis.

- Red and inflamed lids.
- Chemosis of conjunctiva.
- An abscess may form over the upper eyelid.
- Reduction in visual acuity.
- Reduction in colour vision.
- Malaise and fever.
- Relative afferent pupil defect.
- Possible double vision.
- Limitations and painful ocular movements.
- In advanced cases, there may be signs of optic nerve dysfunction.

Patient's needs

- Admission to hospital if necessary.
- All suspected cases of orbital cellulitis will need to have a CT scan to look for any sight/life-threatening subperiosteal and orbital collections. The scan will also show evidence of any adjacent sinus disease. If adjacent sinus disease is not located but intraconal opacity seen on the CT scan, trauma or foreign body should be suspected.
- Relief of symptoms:
  - o   pain – especially on eye movement
  - o   fever – there may be rigors
  - o   anorexia
  - o   general malaise.

Nursing action

- Admit patient to ward if necessary.
- Arrange urgent CT scan of paranasal sinuses orbits and brain.
- Arrange urgent referral to ear, nose and throat specialist.
- Bloods for FBC (full blood count) urea, electrolytes and glucose.
- It is important to liaise with microbiologist, especially if local changes in sensitivity and resistance occur.
- Give prescribed analgesia for pain. Local heat application may be comforting.
- Fan and/or tepid sponge patient to bring down temperature.
- Administer prescribed antibiotics:
  - o   oral, e.g. Clindamycin and Ciprofloxacin – oral antibiotics are normally continued for up to six weeks
  - o   eyedrops, e.g. G. Chloramphenicol, Gentamicin, 2–4 hourly
  - o   in severe cases, intravenous antibiotics may be prescribed.
- Give nourishing fluids and a light diet.
- General nursing care of an ill patient.
- Dress abscess if this forms.
- Prepare for, and give, post-operative care of patient following drainage of abscess sinuses. Send any pus from drainage for sampling.

- Monitoring of optic nerve function hourly – testing visual acuity, pupillary reactions, assessing colour vision using the Ishihara colour vision chart and light brightness appreciation (Kanski, 2003).
- Prolapsed conjunctiva requires a Frost suture and lubricants.

Complications

- The infection may spread backwards into the brain causing:
  - cavernous sinus thrombosis
  - meningitis
  - brain abscess.
- Panophthalmitis may occur.
- Sinus formation, if the cause is a sinusitis.
- Optic atrophy due to pressure on the nerve.
- Subperiorbital abscess.
- Central retinal vein or artery occlusion.
- Raised intra-ocular pressure.
- Exposure keratopathy.

If orbital cellulitis occurs in a child, he is usually referred to an ear, nose and throat specialist, as the cause is invariably from ethmoidal/maxillary sinus.

Preseptal cellulitis

This is infection of the eyelids only, i.e. preseptal. Preseptal cellulitis is often preceded by infection of the teeth or sinuses, by trauma or infected lid chalazion (inflammatory cyst). The infection does not spread beyond the orbital septum of the upper lid into the orbit. The signs and symptoms are similar to orbital cellulitis but the condition is not so dangerous.

If a child presents with obvious lid cyst, treat with oral antibiotics and consider drainage. The child must be reviewed daily until improvement is seen. The child is to be admitted if unwell, if in pain, if it is due to trauma, if no clear history, if parental understanding is poor or if significant ptosis is obstructing examination.

Cavernous sinus thrombosis

The cavernous sinus is situated near the pituitary gland. Through it pass many of the veins draining structures around the face, including the orbit, globe, nose, mouth, sinuses and the meninges. Thus infection can spread from any of these structures into the cavernous sinus. It may also spread from a general infectious disease or septic focus elsewhere in the body. It is a serious condition. Fifty percent of cases are bilateral.

Signs

Signs are as for orbital cellulitis, plus some others:

- paralysis of the extra-ocular muscles, as their nerves pass through the cavernous sinus and are thus involved.
- dilated pupil(s), usually non-reactive due to the trigeminal nerve being involved as it also passes through the cavernous sinus
- anaesthetic cornea due to the involvement of the trigeminal nerve
- reduced visual acuity due to pressure
- papilloedema due to pressure
- signs of cerebral irritation may also be present.

Patient's needs and nursing action

- These are as for orbital cellulitis.
- The antibiotics will be administered by the intravenous route in large doses.
- Anticoagulants may be prescribed.

Thyrotoxic exophthalmos

Graves' disease describes the most common cause of hyperthyroidism and is thought to be due to an autoimmune problem. It usually affects women between the ages of 20 and 45 who have signs and symptoms of thyrotoxicosis together with ophthalmic signs. Ophthalmic signs can occur in patients who are clinically euthyroid and in these cases the disease is referred to as ophthalmic Graves' disease. The signs and symptoms tend to be similar.

Signs

- Exophthalmos – unilateral or bilateral. Inflammatory exudates and plasma cell infiltration of the orbital fat and extra-ocular muscles push the globe forwards (Fig. 5.5).
- Lid lag – when looking downwards, the top lid normally moves with the eye. In this condition, the lid moves very slowly down or not at all. This is possibly due to sympathetic overactivity of Müller's muscle.
- Lid retraction – the upper lid retracts, giving the typical 'stare' associated with thyroid eye disease. The sclera above the cornea is visible. This is probably due to involvement of the levator muscle.
- Corneal exposure – corneal exposure occurs because:
  ○ the lids are unable to close over the protruding globe
  ○ defective blinking occurs because of involvement of the lid muscles.
- Exophthalmoplegia – this is the inability to move the eye in the fields of gaze because the extra-ocular muscles are involved due to infiltration and later fibrosis. Diplopia results.

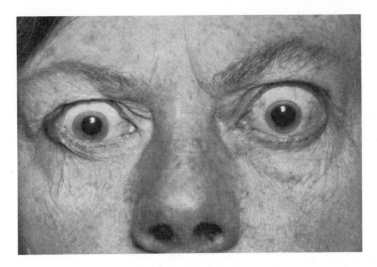

Fig. 5.5 Mild exophthalmos.

- In hyperthyroidism, signs of thyrotoxicosis such as tachycardia and muscular tremors may be present.

Patient's needs

- Protection of the exposed cornea is the most important factor.
- Prevention of complications, which can result in loss of vision.
- Investigation and treatment of thyroid state by an endocrinologist.
- Correction of diplopia.
- Treatment of lid lag.
- In severe cases, rapid relief of orbital pressure.
- Psychological care, the patient may be frightened and in need of reassurance.

Nursing action

- Corneal exposure – the nurse will:
  - instruct the patient in application of ointment such as simple eye ointment or Chloramphenicol at night
  - prepare the patient for a tarsorrhaphy, which may be necessary; the edges of the eyelids are sewn together, usually in the lateral aspect, to protect the cornea
  - instruct the patient in the use and care of a bandage contact lens; this is a large contact lens which covers the whole of the cornea, thereby giving protection (see Appendix 2: Contact Lenses)
- Explain the investigations needed for thyroid function estimations.

- Explain to the patient that diplopia can be treated by wearing glasses with prisms in the lenses. Squint operation may be carried out when the thyroid state is stable.
- Treatment for lid lag – the nurse will prepare the patient for lid surgery when Müller's muscle will be divided.
- In severe cases, where emergency treatment is required to reduce the orbital pressure, the nurse will:
  - give the prescribed high doses of systemic steroids
  - prepare the patient for orbital decompression – part of the lateral wall of the orbit is removed so the orbital contents can prolapse and therefore relieve the pressure on the optic nerve
  - prepare the patient for radiotherapy.

Complications

- Corneal ulceration due to exposure keratitis.
- Visual loss due to optic nerve compression, central retinal artery and vein occlusion.
- Cataract formation due to metabolic disturbance to the lens.
- Secondary glaucoma due to compression on the globe by the orbital contents, causing the intra-ocular pressure to rise.

Conditions of the eyelids

Chalazion

A chalazion is a swelling of one of the Meibomian glands due to a blockage of its duct (Fig. 5.6). It can affect either the upper or lower lid. It may become infected, when it is sometimes called an internal hordeolum. Staphylococci are commonly the cause of the infection. The swelling may fluctuate in size during the course of the condition. Some chalazions point

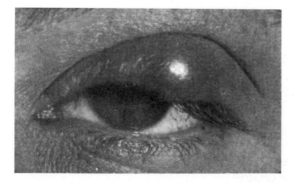

Fig. 5.6 Meibomian cyst.

to the skin surface. Some people appear to be prone to this condition and should be examined to ensure that they are not diabetic. Some chalazions are so large as to obstruct vision and, by pressing on the cornea, cause astigmatism.

Patient's needs

- Relief of swollen eyelid, which is causing pain and discomfort.
- Relief of sticky discharge, which may be present.

Nursing action

- Instruct the patient to apply steam/hot bathing to the eye (see p. 49).
- Instruct the patient in the use of the antibiotic ointment which will be prescribed if the chalazion is infected. Chloramphenicol is the usual ointment. This is used three to four times a day after the eye has been steamed. This should be continued for 14 days.
- Instruct the patient to keep the eyelids clean by, twice a day using warm water to wash off any crusts and discharge.
- Instruct the patient to return if the swelling does not subside, as the simple operation of incision and curettage can be performed once the infection has cleared up, to remove any remaining material.

Oedema of the lids

Oedema of the lids is a common condition and, because of the looseness of the tissue, the swelling can be so great as to close the eye.

Causes

- Insect bites/stings.
- Dermatitis.
- Stye.
- Chalazion.
- Associated with:
  - orbital cellulitis
  - conjunctivitis
  - dacryocystitis
  - drug allergy (Fig. 5.7).

Patient's needs

- Reduction of swelling.
- Treatment of cause.
- Analgesia as required.

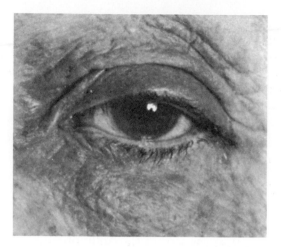

Fig. 5.7 Atopic irritation.

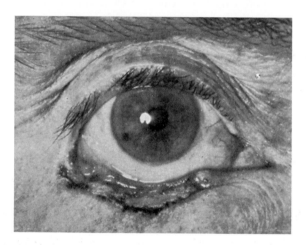

Fig. 5.8 Staphylococcal blepharitis.

Nursing action

- Explain to the patient methods to reduce the swelling:
  - cold compress
  - bathing eyelid with sodium bicarbonate solution
- Explain to him the treatment of the cause of the condition. Antihistamine ointment and/or tablets may be used to treat insect bites/stings.

Blepharitis

Blepharatis can be an acute or a chronic inflammatory condition of the lid margins and is usually bilateral (Fig. 5.8). Blepharitis is often undetected, even when eyes have been examined for other reasons (Bonner et al., 1994).

Causes

- Staphylococcal – chronic infection.
- Seborrhoeic – excessive secretion of lipid from Meibomian glands.
- It may be associated with dandruff, poor hygiene, eczema or allergy to make-up, or drugs.
- Acne rosacea.

Signs

- red, swollen lid margins
- scales on lashes
- eyelid irritation
- burning sensation
- itching
- loss of eye lashes (Schwab et al., 1997).

Patient's needs

- Relief of symptoms:
  - itchiness around eye
  - discharge if an infective cause
  - burning sensation.

Nursing action

- Instruct patient on the treatment:
  - use clean, warm, face cloth over eyelids:
    - (i) Clean lid margin and lashes with diluted baby shampoo or diluted sodium bicarbonate ($\frac{1}{2}$ teaspoon to $\frac{1}{2}$ cup of cooled, boiled water) twice a day. Use good quality cotton buds or wrap a clean face cloth round your first finger
    - (ii) application of antibiotic ointment along the lid margin two or three times a day, if severe
  - dandruff – treatment of dandruff in head hair with antidandruff shampoo
  - make-up – stop using make-up or change the brand used: at the end of the day, remove all traces of make-up (Wittpen, 1995)
  - eczema – may be treated with steroid ointment
  - drugs – stop offending drug
  - poor hygiene – instruct patient on improving general hygiene, especially to hair, face and hands.
- Inform patient that the treatment will need to continue for several weeks, if not for life, as it is a chronic condition although the frequency of treatment can be reduced. Encourage him not to give up the treatment, even if it does not appear to be working in the initial stages.
- Relief of soreness and itching – moisten clean face cloth under hot (as hot as you can stand) running water. Wring it out and place over closed

eyelids. Repeat as the heat goes out of the face cloth (Schwab et al., 1997).

- Patients who are dependent on their carers for their other hygiene needs should also be shown the technique of lid hygiene.

Complications

Complications can occur following blepharitis caused by infective organisms that result in ulceration of the lid margin:

- Conjunctivitis.
- Trichiasis and its sequelae due to chronic ulceration, which, when healed, contract the skin in that area, causing the lash(es) to turn inwards.
- Entropion or ectropion of the lower lid in particular.
- Corneal ulcer.

Stye or external hordeolum

A stye or external hordeolum is an inflammation of a gland of Zeis that opens into the lash follicle. An abscess forms, which usually points near an eyelash (Fig. 5.9).

Signs

- Swelling, often with pointing on the lid margin situated near a lash.

Patient's needs

- Relief of pain and swelling.

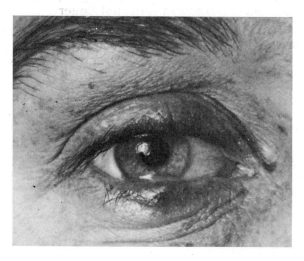

Fig. 5.9 An external stye.

Nursing action

- Explain the treatment, which is similar to that for a chalazion (see p. 68).
- Incision and curettage is not necessary for a stye. Removal of the affected lash will cause the abscess to drain, but this action is momentarily very painful.
- If styes recur, the patient should be investigated for diabetes mellitus.

Trichiasis

Trichiasis is a condition in which the lashes grow inwards and rub on the cornea. This may follow, for example, blepharitis, trauma or surgery to the lids. Often the cause is unknown.

Patient's needs

- Removal of the offending lash(es) which is(are) causing irritation to the eye.

Nursing action

- Remove the lash by:
  - epilating it using epilation forceps (see p. 33); this will need to be repeated regularly
  - assisting the doctor or specialist nurse to use electrolysis, when an electrode is introduced to each offending lash follicle to destroy it:
    - (i)   prepare local anaesthetic injection and drops
    - (ii)   instil antibiotic ointment to the eye following the procedure
  - assisting the doctor to apply cryotherapy (liquid nitrogen) to the lash follicle to destroy it:
    - (i)   prepare local anaesthetic injection and drops
    - (ii)   instil antibiotic ointment following the procedure
    - (iii)   warn the patient that the eye will be uncomfortable for a few days following cryotherapy
  - assisting the doctor to apply argon laser (Yung et al., 1994) to the offending lash.
- Check the cornea for abrasions from the ingrowing lash(es) by staining lashes with G. Fluorescein. If abrasions have occurred, instruct the patient to use the prescribed antibiotic ointment three times a day for three or four days.
- Instruct the patient to return for further lash epilation as soon as he feels that the eye is becoming irritated, so that complications can be avoided by prompt treatment.

Complications

- Corneal abrasions.
- Corneal ulceration.
- Superficial corneal opacities.
- Vascularisation of the cornea.
- Unfortunately, treatment is rarely completely successful and usually needs to be repeated at regular intervals.

Entropion

Entropion is the turning inwards of the eyelid, usually the lower lid (Fig. 5.10).

Causes

- Spastic entropion occurring in old age when spasm of the orbicularis muscle occurs, causing the lid to turn inwards.
- Cicatricial contraction of the palpebral conjunctiva following trauma or disease to the lid or conjunctiva.

Patient's needs

- Relief of symptoms of irritation in the eye.

Nursing action

- Strap the lower lid to pull it outwards (see p. 38).
- Prepare the patient and equipment for surgery to evert the lid. Care must be taken when performing entropion surgery to avoid an ectropion resulting.
- Entropion operations include:
  - cautery
  - transverse lid everting suture

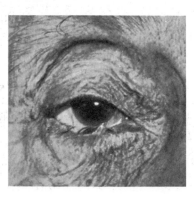

Fig. 5.10 Spastic entropion.

- o   Wies procedure – lid splitting and marginal rotation
- o   Fox procedure – excision of triangle of conjunctiva and tarsal plate
- o   shortening of lower lid retractors.

Complications

- The complications for entropion are the same as those for trichiasis.

Ectropion

Ectropion is the turning outwards of the eyelid, usually the lower lid (Fig. 5.11).

Causes

- Senile ectropion due to relaxation of the orbicularis muscle, turning the eyelid outwards.
- Cicatricial ectropion due to scarring following trauma or chronic disease of the lid or conjunctiva, pulling lid outwards.
- Paralytic ectropion occurring with palsies of the seventh cranial nerve.

Because the punctum is not in apposition to the bulbar conjunctiva when an ectropion is present, the tears cannot flow through the punctum and into the lacrimal drainage system. They therefore spill over the lid margin and down the cheek.

Patient's needs

- Relief of symptoms:
  - o   watering eye
  - o   irritable sensation
  - o   discharge, which may be present
  - o   sore skin area over maxilla from constantly wiping away tears.

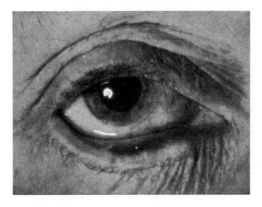

Fig. 5.11 Ectropion.

Nursing action

- Prepare the patient and equipment for surgery to invert the lid:
  - lazy-T procedure – full thickness excision
  - retropunctal cautery
  - Bick procedure – full thickness excision.

Care must be taken when performing ectropion surgery to avoid an entropion resulting.

Ptosis

Ptosis is drooping of the upper lid. It may be unilateral, bilateral, constant or intermittent.

Causes

- Congenital ptosis (Fig. 5.12) is caused by failure of development of the levator muscle. It is usually bilateral. The child with bilateral congenital ptosis has to tilt his head backwards to be able to see properly. This will prevent amblyopia developing (see p. 189). There is a danger that amblyopia will occur with unilateral ptosis.
- Acquired ptosis is caused by:
  - mechanical failure – abnormal weight on lid due to oedema, tumour, scarring
  - muscle involvement – trauma to muscle. Disease involving muscles, e.g. muscular dystrophy, myasthenia gravis. If, following an injection of neostigmine, the ptosis is temporarily relieved, myasthenia can be diagnosed
  - paralysis of nerves supplying the upper lid.

Patient's needs

- Correction of lid, if it obscures sight.
- Treatment of underlying disease.

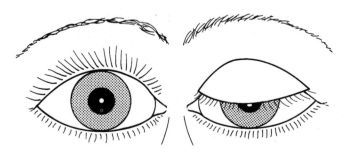

Fig. 5.12 Left ptosis.

Nursing action

- Explain and prepare the patient for any of the following treatments:
  - lid surgery to resect the levator muscle or remove growths if present
  - wearing of special glasses or contact lenses with 'ptosis edge' to hold the lid up
  - treatment of causative or underlying disease, e.g. myasthenia gravis.

Bell's palsy

Bell's palsy is due to paralysis of the seventh nerve with resulting incomplete lids closure and corneal exposure. As a result of ineffective lid closure and corneal exposure, patients may present with a painful, red watery eye. The early management of Bell's palsy is aimed at the painful red eye. Initially copious topical lubricant and taping of the eyelid at night is all that is required. The patient will need constant reassurance and support at every stage. If corneal exposure is severe, a temporary lateral tarsorrhaphy may be needed. Lateral tarsorrhaphy joins the upper and lower lids laterally in order to reduce the palpebral aperture and protect the cornea. The long-term management of poor lid closure may include the implantation of gold weights into the upper lid. This procedure allows a better lid closure and a more natural blink. Possible complications may include extrusion or migration (Collin & Rose, 2001).

Blepharospasm

This is a condition that causes forceful, painful spasm eyelid closure resulting in difficulty in opening the eye. Photophobia is present and the condition is exacerbated by bright lights, stress and excessive movement around the person. It can cause the individual concerned to become socially isolated and unable to work. There may be some accompanying contraction of the lower facial muscles. Treatment is by injections of Botulinum (Osaka & Keltner, 1991) into the orbicularis muscle. This is repeated every two to three months.

Tumours

Growths on the eyelids can be either benign or malignant.

Benign

- Papilloma.
- Warts.
- Granulomas.
- Xanthelasma.

Malignant

- Basal cell carcinoma (see Colour Plates 6 and 7).
- Squamous cell carcinoma.
- Melanoma.

Patient's needs

- Removal of tumour, especially if it is thought to be malignant.
- Mohs' micrographic surgery (where available) is used in the management of periocular basal cell carcinoma. Mohs' micrographic surgery allows each cancerous layer to be visualised through the microscope. Excision of the cancerous layer continues until cancer-free layers are obtained.

Nursing action

- Prepare the patient and equipment for removal of the tumour. Skin grafting or flaps may be necessary depending on the size and position of the tumour.
- Send specimen to the laboratory for histology.

Surgery to the lids must be performed with great care to avoid either an ectropion, entropion or trichiasis resulting.

Chapter 6
The Lacrimal System and Tear Film

Introduction

The lacrimal system (Fig. 6.1) consists of:

- the lacrimal gland
- the lacrimal drainage system comprising:
  - the puncta
  - the canaliculi
  - the lacrimal sac
  - the nasolacrimal duct.

The lacrimal gland

The lacrimal gland is situated in the upper, outer quadrant of the orbit, in the lacrimal fossa of the frontal bone. It is almond-shaped and is divided into two lobes by the levator palpebral muscle:

- the superior or orbital lobe
- the inferior or palpebral lobe.

There are 10 to 12 drainage channels leaving the lacrimal gland to convey tears to openings in the upper fornix.

Blood supply

The lacrimal artery and vein supply and drain blood to and from the lacrimal gland.

Nerve supply

Nerve supply to the lacrimal gland is via the lacrimal nerve, the first branch of the ophthalmic division of the trigeminal nerve.

Function of the lacrimal gland

The function of the lacrimal gland is to produce tears in response to stimulation of the trigeminal nerve through, for example, emotion; foreign body

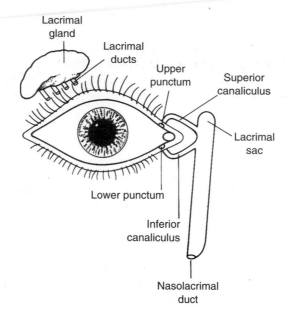

Fig. 6.1 Lacrimal system. (Reprinted from Darling & Thorpe *Ophthalmic Nursing* (1981), Fig. 36, p. 144 by permission of the publisher Baillière Tindall Limited, London.)

on the cornea or conjunctiva; or noxious fumes, such as smoke or peeled onions.

The lacrimal drainage system

The puncta

The upper and lower puncta are small round or slightly oval apertures situated on the lid margin on a slight elevation called the lacrimal papilla. This is a pale area, due to the presence of few blood vessels, about 6 mm from the inner canthus. Both puncta are normally turned inwards towards the bulbar conjunctiva so tears can drain into them. Fibres of the orbicularis muscle surround them.

The canaliculi

The upper and lower canaliculi are narrow ducts passing from each puncta vertically for 1.5–2.0 mm, which then turn medially and travel horizontally for 10 mm. They usually unite to form a common canaliculus for about 1 mm before opening out into the lacrimal sac.

The lacrimal sac

The lacrimal sac is situated in the lacrimal fossa of the lacrimal bone. It is blind-ended superiorly, 5 mm wide and 12–14 mm in length. Fibres of the orbicularis and Horner's muscles surround the sac.

The nasolacrimal duct

The nasolacrimal duct is a downward continuation of the sac for 12–24 mm before opening into the inferior meatus of the nose beneath the inferior turbinate bone. The valve of Hasner, a mucosal fold, covers part of the opening. All the passages of the lacrimal drainage system are lined with epithelium.

Blood supply

Blood is supplied to the nasolacrimal duct via the nasal artery and the superior and inferior medial palpebral artery. Drainage is via the nasal vein and the superior and inferior medial palpebral veins.

Nerve supply

The infratrochlear nerve, a branch of the nasociliary nerve, which is the third branch of the ophthalmic division of the trigeminal nerve, provides the nerve supply for the nasolacrimal duct.

Lymphatic drainage

Lymph is drained from the nasolacrimal duct via the submaxillary nodes.

The tear film

The tear film is a mixture of secretions from the accessory tear glands of Krause and Wolfring, the goblets cells of the conjunctiva and the Meibomian glands of the eyelids. The tear film is a constant film of fluid bathing the conjunctiva and cornea. The lacrimal gland produces excess tears.

Three layers of the tear film

These layers are illustrated in Fig. 6.2:

(1) Oil: the outer layer, produced by the Meibomian glands of the tarsal plates and also the glands of Moll and Zeis. The oily layer prevents evaporation and spillage of tears over the lid margin.
(2) Aqueous: the middle layer, the 'tears proper', produced by the lacrimal gland and the glands of Krause and Wolfring.
(3) Mucin: the inner layer, produced by the goblet cells of the conjunctiva, is a wetting substance for easy spread over the cornea.

Composition of tears

- 98% water
- 2–5% protein

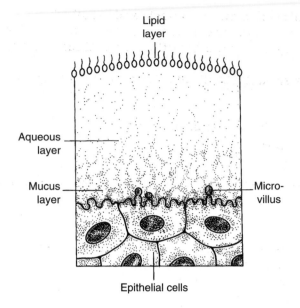

Fig. 6.2 Three layers of the tear film. (Reproduced with permission from Vaughan, D.G. & Asbury, T. (1983) *General Ophthalmology* (10th edn), Appleton & Lange.)

- Glucose
- Urea
- Sodium
- Potassium
- Retinol
- Chloride
- Lysozyme – an antimicrobial enzyme
- Immunoproteins and antimicrobial agents
- Normal pH is between 6.5–7.6 (Forrester et al., 2002).

Function of tears

- Refraction – to provide an optically smooth surface to the cornea.
- Lubrication of the front of the eyeball.
- Cleansing action by washing away dust particles from the eye.
- Protection from infection by secreting the enzyme lysozyme and immunoproteins and antimicrobial agents.

Flow of tears

Tears flow across the front of the eyeball into the lacrimal drainage channels as a result of the following factors:

- Gravity itself assists tear flow.
- Blinking: lid movements assist the flow of tears across the front of the cornea and conjunctiva.

- Capillary attraction into the puncta and canaliculi.
- The lacrimal pump: the contraction of orbicularis and Horner's muscles around the puncta and lacrimal sac dilate these structures and draw in the tears.
- Some tears are lost as a result of evaporation into the atmosphere.

Conditions of the lacrimal system

Dacryoadenitis

Dacryoadenitis is a rare acute or chronic inflammation of the lacrimal gland. Causes include:

- Acute:
  - complication of systemic infections such as: mumps, measles, infectious mononucleosis or influenza
  - trachoma
  - herpes zoster
  - staphylococcal infection
  - following injury to the lacrimal gland.
- Chronic:
  - sarcoidosis
  - tuberculosis
  - syphilis
  - lymphatic leukaemia
  - lymphosarcoma.

Signs and symptoms

Acute:

- Pain: swelling and redness of the upper lid, especially in the upper temporal aspect (Fig. 6.3).
- S-shaped curve to the upper lid.

Patient's needs

- Relief of pain must be a priority.
- Admission to hospital may be necessary if condition is severe.
- Incision of abscess where necessary.
- Application of warm compresses (as hot as the patient can tolerate without causing heat trauma) can provide some relief.
- Treatment of active infection with appropriate antibiotic.
- Treatment of underlying cause, if possible.

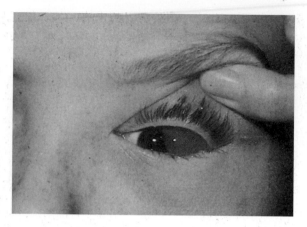

Fig. 6.3 Dacryoadenitis.

Nursing action

- Admit patient to hospital if condition is severe.
- Give/advise the patient:
  - to instil antibiotic drops and ointment, usually for 7–10 days
  - to take any prescribed oral antibiotics for the duration of the course
  - to take analgesics or apply local heat for pain relief.
- Prepare patient and equipment for incision of abscess.
- Chronic: Normally painless and develops slowly. Treatment is usually with warm compresses and antibiotic therapy.

Dacryocystitis

Dacryocystitis is an acute or chronic inflammation of the lacrimal sac (Fig. 6.4). It is a rare condition but more common than dacryoadenitis. It is usually unilateral and is associated with obstruction to the lacrimal drainage system.

Causes

Acute

- most are unknown
- following chronic dacryocystitis
- causative organisms – *Staphylococci, Streptococci, Pneumococci.*

Chronic

- following trauma to the lacrimal system
- following chronic conjunctivitis, e.g. trachoma.

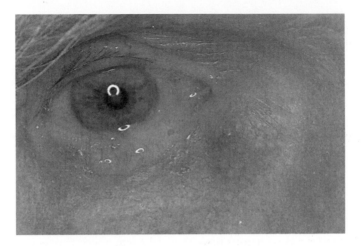

Fig. 6.4 Dacryocystitis.

Infant

Failure of canalisation of lacrimal ducts following birth.

Signs

Adult acute and infant:

- pain
- red, tender swelling over lacrimal sac
- pus regurgitating through punctum
- conjunctivitis
- watering eye (epiphora) which may cause visual disturbance.

Chronic:

- may be swelling over lacrimal sac, which can be recurrent
- pus may emerge from the punctum when pressure is applied to the sac
- epiphora, which may cause visual disturbance.

Patient's needs

Acute

- relief of pain, which can be severe, with appropriate analgesia; warm compresses can effect some relief of pain
- lid hygiene to address problem of discharge and watering eye.

Chronic

- relief of watering eye due to blockage of drainage channels
- diagnosis and treatment of obstruction.

Infant

- relief of pain
- lid hygiene to address problem of discharge and watering eye
- admission to hospital for probing of ducts if initial treatment fails.

Nursing action

Acute adult

- Apply/instruct the patient how to apply warm compress to the inflamed area (clean face cloths rinsed under a warm tap can provide some relief).
- Give/instruct him to take the prescribed analgesia and antibiotics, e.g. Augmentin 350 mg three times a day for 7–10 days.
- Clean/instruct him how to clean the eye if sticky and instil prescribed antibiotic drops and ointment, usually Chloramphenicol or Fucithalmic.

Chronic adult

- Perform lacrimal sac washout to detect area of blockage (see p. 41). Note: this is never carried out on a patient with an acute infection of the sac as the inflamed walls are easy to perforate.
- Prepare patient for dacryocystogram. This is an X-ray using radio-opaque dye, which is introduced into the lacrimal drainage system to show up any blockage. Warn the patient that it is an uncomfortable procedure and that he should be accompanied home following this test as he may feel unwell.
- Admit and prepare the patient for surgery to correct the blockage. Dacryocystorhinostomy(DCR) is performed to open up a new drainage channel into the nasal cavity. This may be performed using an endoscope or a more traditional external approach through the skin. Sometimes a tube is left in situ (DCR and tubes) for 3–6 months to maintain the patency of the new drainage channels. These tubes should not interfere with the cornea unless they extrude.

Post-operative care

- In the immediate post-operative period, the patient must be monitored carefully for any epistaxis (nosebleed). Blood loss from this can be catastrophic. The haemorrhage may be overt or could be via the back of the throat.
- A pressure dressing will remain in place until the dressing the morning after surgery. This should be observed for signs of haemorrhage.

- In the case of endoscopic DCR, a nasal pack will be in situ. This too must be observed for haemorrhage. It usually is removed the next day.
- Standard DCR:
  - Clean the eye and suture line.
  - Instil antibiotic drops; occasionally antibiotic cream is prescribed to be applied to the suture line. The surgeon may recommend that this is gently massaged in to reduce scarring.
  - Remove sutures 5–7 days post-operatively (usually in out-patient department).
  - Instruct the patient not to blow his nose vigorously as this could cause bleeding and will dislodge the tubing.
  - If a tube is present, it will be removed in the outpatient department. The procedure is relatively painless and does not warrant surgery (see p. 46).

Infant

- Instruct the parent/guardian to instil topical antibiotic drops, e.g. G. Chloramphenicol.
- Instruct the parent/guardian to massage over the lacrimal sac area to remove the accumulated mucus, which may lead to a patent duct.
- Admitting the child to hospital should be considered if these methods fail to open the canaliculus.
- A thorough pre-operative assessment as well as review by the anaesthetist should be completed. Parental or legal guardian's consent must be obtained.
- Probing of the tear ducts will be done under general anaesthetic.
- Give standard pre-operative care prior to probing of the ducts.
- Give post-operative care: instil antibiotic drops.

Complications

Following acute dacryocystitis, fistula formation may develop. Dacryocystorhinostomy is not always successful in curing the watering eye.

Epiphora

Epiphora is watering of the eye (increased lacrimation).

Causes

Causes include:

- acute or chronic dacryocystitis (see above)
- ectropion (see p. 75)
- a small, tight or absent punctum

- increased secretion of tears due to reflex stimulation of the lacrimal gland, e.g. by wind, smoke, onions, or a foreign body in the eye
- allergy, e.g. hay fever.

Patient's needs

- explanation of the condition, its cause and prognosis
- dilation of a small or tight punctum
- removal of causative agent of increased stimulation
- treat hay fever.

Nursing action

- Careful history of the presenting complaint, systematic examination of the eyelids, conjunctiva and the cornea.
- If a foreign body is present, remove this (see p. 36).
- If the cause is a small or tight punctum, this needs to be dilated regularly over a period of several months. This is usually performed every week or so using for example, a Nettleships dilator, holding it in place in the punctum for five minutes.
- Prepare patient and equipment for a one, two or three-snip operation, which will be carried out if the dilation fails. During this procedure, performed under local anaesthetic, snips are made behind the punctum to release the muscle around the punctum.
- Prescribe topical antihistamine drops such as Lodoxamide.

Dry eye syndrome (keratoconjunctivitis sicca)

Dryness of the eye results from any disease associated with deficiency of any of the layers of the tear film as well as lid or corneal surface abnormalities. Its name (dry eyes) implies a non-significant condition. This is not the case. In addition to being very uncomfortable, it has the potential to be sight threatening.

Causes

- lacrimal gland failure
- oil deficiency
- exposure: proptosis, facial palsy
- hot, dry climate/environment
- lid damage
- blepharitis
- meibomianitis
- aqueous deficiency
- Sjögren's syndrome (arthritis, dry eye, achlorhydria)
- removal/absence of glands
- trachoma

- chronic dacryoadenitis
- drugs: beta-blockers, diuretics
- old age
- menopause
- mucin deficiency
- chemical burns
- chronic conjunctivitis
- antihistamines
- Stevens-Johnson syndrome
- xerophthalmia.
- other causes: deficient blinking; corneal scarring.

Signs

- Usually a normal-looking eye.
- Damaged epithelial, corneal and conjunctival cells stain with fluorescein drops.
- Breaks in the tear film are seen when stained with G. Fluorescein. The normal tear break-up time is usually over ten seconds.

Patient's needs

- An adequate explanation of the condition.
- Recognition that it causes ocular disturbance.
- Advice that this is a chronic condition and treatment is about relieving symptoms or preventing symptoms occurring.
- Relief of symptoms that include:
  - gritty feeling
  - itching
  - burning sensation
  - inability to produce tears
  - pain around and in the eye
  - sometimes a red eye
  - difficulty in opening eyes on waking and moving lids
  - excessive watering eye (if the outer oil layer of the tear film is deficient, tears will spill over the lower lid margin).
- Investigation and treatment of underlying cause, if possible.
- Treatment with replacement tears.

Nursing action

- Perform tear production test (see p. 38).
- Instruct the patient to use the prescribed artificial tears, e.g. hypromellose. These drops can usually be used as often as the patient requires, keeping the eye feeling comfortable, and will probably need long-term use.

- Cautery to the punctum or insertion of punctal plugs may be employed to prevent what little tears are produced from draining into the punctum.

Complications

- Chronic conjunctivitis due to loss of the protective function of the tear film and lysozyme.
- Corneal scarring and vascularisation.
- Corneal ulceration, thinning and perforation.
- Eventual loss of the eye through recurrent infections.

Chapter 7
The Conjunctiva

Introduction

The conjunctiva is a thin, transparent mucous membrane lining the upper and lower lids and covering the globe up to the limbus.

Areas of the conjunctiva

There are three areas to the conjunctiva:

- Palpebral conjunctiva – lines the upper and lower lids.
- Bulbar conjunctiva – reflects back to cover the sclera up to the limbus.
- Fornices – the upper and lower fornices are blind sacs, formed where the bulbar and palpebral conjunctiva fold back over each other.

Layers of the conjunctiva

The epithelial layer contains the goblet cells; the stromal layer contains the blood vessels, nerves and the glands of Krause and Wolfring (in upper only).

The conjunctiva is connected to Tenon's Capsule around the limbus. Elsewhere it is loosely attached, especially in the fornices where there are folds of the conjunctiva. This allows for easy mobility of the eyeball.

Functions of the conjunctiva

- Allows easy movement of the eyeball.
- Goblet cells provide mucin for the tear film.
- It is a protective layer to the eyeball by being a physical barrier and by its rich blood supply.

Blood supply

There is a rich blood supply, especially in the fornices, delivered and drained via:

- anterior ciliary artery and vein
- superior and inferior medial palpebral artery and vein
- conjunctival artery and vein.

Nerve supply

The nerve supply to the conjunctiva is by the long ciliary branch of the nasociliary nerve from the trigeminal nerve.

Lymphatic drainage

Lymphatic drainage is through the pre-auricular, parotid and submaxillary nodes.

Conditions of the conjunctiva

Conjunctivitis

Conjunctivitis is inflammation of the conjunctiva, which has several causes:

- bacterial
- viral
- allergic
- chlamydial
- fungal
- parasitic
- associated with other diseases
- other ophthalmic conditions
- mechanical.

Bacterial conjunctivitis

Bacterial conjunctivitis can be either acute or chronic.

Causative organisms

- *Streptococcus.*
- *Staphylococcus aureus.*
- *Pneumococcus.*
- *Gonococcus.*
- *Haemolytic Streptococcus.*

Signs

Typically there is conjunctival injection, especially in the fornices where the blood supply is rich (Fig. 7.1). The eye may, on the other hand, be white or only mildly red. Discharge is variable, but typically is present in the mornings, and on waking the eye is difficult to open because the eyelids are stuck together. This is a very important point when taking a history from a patient with suspected conjunctivitis. The eyelids may be red and inflamed. The condition may be unilateral or bilateral. The vision is always unaffected and

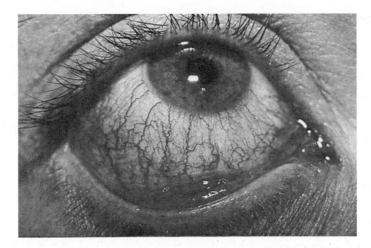

Fig. 7.1 Bacterial conjunctivitis. (Reproduced with permission from Khaw, P.T. & Elkington, A.R. (1985) Disorders of the external eye, *The Practitioner*, **229**, 317.)

there is usually no pain. The patient may complain of a gritty or foreign body sensation, some discomfort and very occasionally very mild photophobia.

Nursing action

- Check the patient's visual acuity.
- Swabs are only necessary if there is any doubt of the diagnosis or if the condition has not resolved.
- Obtain an accurate history from patient to determine a correct diagnosis.
- Examination of the eye on slit lamp to confirm diagnosis
- Clean the eye(s) and instruct the patient on cleaning it (them), using cooled, boiled water.
- Give verbal and written instruction on how to instil the eye drops. This is usually Chloramphenicol drops, which may be prescribed four times a day for a period of 7–10 days. In severe cases, Chloramphenicol drops may be prescribed every two hours for two days and then four times a day for 7–10 days. If warranted, an ointment can also be prescribed for night-time application. In order to reduce the risk of complication arising from the use of chloramphenicol drops, it is advisable to check for any family/history of blood disorder since there have been reported cases of aplastic anaemia (Field, Martin & Witchell, 1999). Caution should also be exercised in women who are pregnant. If in doubt, Fucidic Acid (Fucithalmic) can be prescribed instead. In children, it is wise to prescribe Fucidic Acid as this only necessitates a twice-daily drop regime.
- Instruct patient on how to prevent the spread of infection either to his other eye or to other members of the household:
  - Wash hands before and after instilling eye medications.

    ○ Use separate face flannels and towels in the home, as this is the usual method of spread of infection. Change face flannels and towels daily.

    ○ Use clean tissues rather than handkerchief to reduce the spread of infection.

    ○ Change pillowcases daily.

- Keep Chloramphenicol drops in a cool place, preferably in a fridge.
- Never share drops and ointment with anyone else.
- It is important that patients are reminded to finish all the prescribed course of treatment.
- Warn him not to wear a pad over the eye, as it provides a suitable environment for a further bacterial growth.
- If eye make-up is used, advise the patient to discard and buy new cosmetics when infection has cleared up.

Ophthalmia neonatorum

Severe conjunctivitis occurring in a baby less than 28 days old is a notifiable disease. This may be caused by *Gonococcus*, *Streptococcus*, or *Chlamydia* which is the most common cause. However, this condition needs to be distinguished from the neonatal conjunctivitis caused by nasolacrimal obstruction with other bacterial infection, trauma and inclusion conjunctivitis agents.

Signs

- severe discharge
- red, swollen eyelids (Fig. 7.2)
- chemosis
- unilateral or bilateral infection.

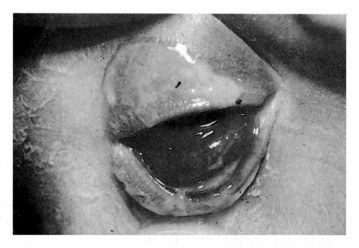

Fig. 7.2 Ophthalmia neonatorum.

Nursing action

- The condition must be clearly and sensitively explained to both parents (or carers). They should be told of the baby's diagnosis and the likelihood of how the baby has the infection.
- Both parents must be screened and examined at the genito-urinary medicine clinic.
- Clean/instruct the parent to instil the prescribed antibiotics.
- Topical Tetracycline is the treatment of choice.
- This condition can be associated with Otitis media and gastrointestinal tract infections so oral antibiotics are usually prescribed.

Complications of chronic conjunctivitis

- conjunctival scarring
- chronic blepharitis due to upset in the tear film
- conjunctival ulceration leading to perforation due to decreased conjunctival nutrition
- marginal corneal ulcer.

Viral conjunctivitis

Causes

- Adenovirus
- Measles
- Varicella
- Herpes simplex (see p. 108)
- *Chlamydia.*

Signs

- red/pink eye (Fig. 7.3)
- chemosis, if severe
- follicles may be present on the palpebral conjunctiva
- cornea – superficial punctate keratitis
- enlarged pre-auricular nodes, which may be tender
- bleeding from conjunctival vessels in severe adenoviral conjunctivitis.

Patient's needs

- Relief of symptoms:
  - watering eye
  - irritation, which may be present
  - photophobia
  - generally unwell feeling.
- Instruction on treatment.

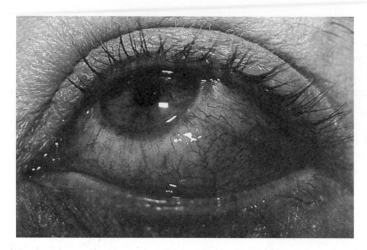

Fig. 7.3 Adenoviral conjunctivitis. (Reproduced with permission from Khaw, P.T. & Elkington, A.R.(1985) Disorders of the external eye, *The Practitioner*, **229**, 317.)

Nursing action

- Treatment is mainly supportive and educative since there is no effective treatment for adenovirus conjunctivitis.
- Usually no treatment is given as viral infections are self-limiting, running a course of 7–10 days.
- Artificial lubricant can be prescribed for patient comfort.
- Full explanation of the condition to increase patient awareness and reduce discomfort.
- General advice for hygiene is the same as for bacterial conjunctivitis.
- Thorough cleaning of slit lamps using HAZ or Milton solutions.
- If prisms are used during the examination, where possible, use disposable tonoshield or tonosafe. If these are unavailable, then the prism must be wiped clean while moist before the face of the lens is immersed in the disinfection fluid normally used. At the end of each clinic session, the prisms should be cleaned with detergent, rinsed thoroughly in sterile saline and then wiped dry (RCO guidelines, 2002).
- Vigilant hand washing by all medical and nursing personnel.
- If photophobia is present, advise patient to wear dark glasses.

Allergic conjunctivitis

Causes

- hay fever – tends to be seasonal.

Signs

- severe chemosis
- red eye
- papillae may be present on the palpebral conjunctiva.

Symptoms

- irritation of the eye
- watering eye
- nasal signs of hay fever may be present.

Treatment

- antihistamines such as Xylometazoline Hydrochloride (Otrivine Antisin) drops four times a day or
- G. Sodium Cromoglycate (Opticron) 2% four times a day
- steroids, if condition is severe.

Vernal conjunctivitis or spring catarrh

A common seasonal, warm-weather condition, some patients being affected annually in the spring or early summer (see Fig. 7.4). It usually affects the 10–14 years age group, boys more than girls.

Signs

- giant papillae on subtarsal conjunctiva, called 'cobblestones' (see Colour Plate 1)
- corneal punctate epithelial erosions.

Symptoms

- irritation, foreign body sensation in the eye

Treatment

- G. Sodium Cromoglycate 2%; steroids, if severe
- test for allergy and avoid cause, if possible.

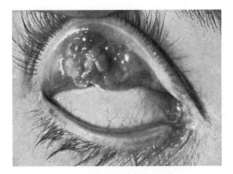

Fig. 7.4 spring catarrh.

Eczema

Signs

- redness of eye
- red, dry, scaly eyelid
- skin around eye may be affected
- slight discharge may be present
- fine papillae on palpebral conjunctiva.

Symptoms

- burning sensation
- photophobia.

Treatment

- antibiotic drops to prevent secondary infection
- steroid cream, e.g. betamethasone or sodium phosphate or hydrocortisone to eyelid and affected skin around the eye.

Chlamydia trachomatis/adult inclusion conjunctivitis

Chlamydia or adult inclusion conjunctivitis is caused by serotypes D to K. It typically affects young adults, with eye symptoms appearing a week after sexual activity. It is important to obtain an accurate history from patient and this should include duration of eye problems, any systemic symptoms, any known sexual contact and any treatment for sexually transmitted disease.

Signs

- red eye
- discharge
- follicles and papillae on palpebral conjunctiva
- chemosis of bulbar conjunctiva
- small tender pre-auricular nodes
- keratitis
- pannus formation on upper portion of the cornea; this is the development of new blood vessels growing into the cornea and is usually a later sign of the disease.

Patient's needs

- Relief of symptoms, pain, photophobia, watering eye.
- Instruction on treatment.

Nursing action

- Take swab for testing for *Chlamydia* ensuring sufficient material is obtained (see p. 27).

- Instruct the patient on the treatment:
  - Oc. chlortetracycline 1% four times a day for six weeks
  - oral tetracycline 250 mg four times a day for six weeks
  - sulphonamides may also be given.
- Sensitivity and tact must be shown to the patients and their partners when informing them of the diagnosis.
- Importance of treating the partners even though they maybe asymptomatic.
- Appointment must be made for them to attend the genito-urinary medicine clinic

Trachoma

Trachoma also known as Egyptian ophthalmia or granular conjunctivitis is caused by an organism called *Chlamydia trachomatis* which is a parasite closely related to bacteria. Trachoma is caused by serotypes A, Ba, C. It is common in hot, dry climates where there is a low standard of hygiene and flies are abundant. The disease runs a long and chronic course. The incubation period is 5–14 days. In a child, the onset is insidious, but it is acute in an adult.

Signs and symptoms

- oedematous eyelids
- discharge
- pain
- follicles especially on upper lid
- photophobia
- repeated attacks leading to entropion and corneal involvement
- long term – corneal scarring leading to severe loss of vision and blindness.

Treatment

- Early stages – antibiotic treatment of tetracyclines, erythromycin or sulphonamides for four to six weeks.

Complications

- Conjunctival scarring and fibrosis resulting in:
  - blockage to the drainage of the accessory tear glands and lacrimal gland resulting in a reduced tear film
  - reduction in secretion of mucin.

Both these results will cause a reduction in lysozyme in the tear film and therefore the patient will be prone to chronic conjunctivitis

- o blocked lacrimal ducts from conjunctival scarring, which could cause dacryocystitis
    - o entropion and trichiasis
    - o ptosis, due to scarring under the top lid.
- Scarring of the cornea due to pannus formation, trichiasis and scarred palpebral conjunctiva.

Treatment of the complications

- Scarred conjunctival tissue can be treated by expressing and curetting the follicles. Plastic surgery may be necessary to correct lid deformities.
- Corneal graft to replace the scarred cornea. This can only be performed once the lid deformities have been corrected so that they will not abrade the grafted cornea.
- Administration of replacement teardrops to treat the dry eyes.
- Use of antibiotic drops for chronic bacterial conjunctivitis.
- Antibiotic treatment for dacryocystitis.
- A dacryocystorhinostomy to correct the blocked nasolacrimal ducts.

Fungal conjunctivitis

Fungal conjunctivitis is caused by *Candida albicans*. Babies can be affected during birth through an infected birth canal. Fine white plaques are apparent on the conjunctiva. Affected adults have blepharitis.

The treatment is with nystatin drops and ointment.

Parasitic conjunctivitis

In hot climates, parasites causing onchoceriasis (river blindness) and schistosomiasis (bilharzia) can induce conjunctivitis.

Conjunctivitis caused by other diseases

General diseases which cause conjunctivitis are:

- skin diseases: psoriasis, pemphygoid, acne rosacea and pemphigus
- Sjögren's syndrome (p. 88)
- thyroid disease
- Reiter's syndrome.

Ophthalmic conditions causing conjunctivitis

- dacryocystitis
- canaliculitis
- dry eyes.

The treatment is that of the general disease or ophthalmic condition.

Mechanical conjunctivitis

Conjunctivitis can occur after the conjunctiva has been exposed to:

- wind
- fumes
- smoke
- dust
- dirt particles
- chemicals.

Subconjunctival haemorrhage

Subconjunctival haemorrhage occurs as a result of blunt or penetrating injury (see Chapter 14) but it can also occur spontaneously or as a result of a sudden increase in pressure in the eye, as occurs with violent sneezing or heavy lifting. The subconjunctival blood vessels burst, with the affected area varying in size; in severe cases the haemorrhage can cover the whole of the sclera causing swelling but usually sparing the superior aspect as it pools inferiorly from gravity. In cases occurring spontaneously, the patients usually have few symptoms apart from a dull ache. It is a condition that looks more severe than it is. It can be a sign of hypertension, vascular disease or a blood clotting disorder.

Patient's needs

- Location of the cause, if any, of spontaneous haemorrhage.

Nursing action

- Ask the patient if he had exerted any undue pressure before the haemorrhage occurred, e.g. by heavy digging in the garden, sneezing fit, rubbing the eye.
- Take the blood pressure; if abnormal, inform the doctor.
- Reassure the patient that the haemorrhage will not cover the cornea.
- Inform him that it may spread further before it begins to resolve and that it may take two to three weeks to clear completely, similar to a bruise. Usually there is no specific treatment.
- Check if patients are on Aspirin, Warfarin or any other relevant medication.
- Advise patient to see GP for advice such as INR check if appropriate.
- If sub-conjunctival haemorrhage is as a result of trauma, the eye has to be carefully examined under the slit lamp for any other injuries.

Pterygium

A pterygium is a triangular-shaped nodule in the conjunctiva (Fig. 7.5), usually occurring on the nasal side, but it can be temporal. It usually occurs

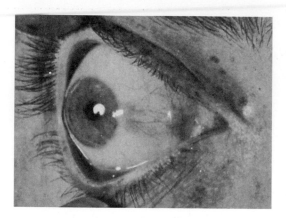

Fig. 7.5 Pterygium.

in people who live in hot, dry climates or who work in the open air. It is a degenerative process and can encroach on the cornea. If it affects the vision, it can be removed under local anaesthetic. Beta rays or cytotoxic eyedrops can be given following removal to prevent recurrence.

Pinguecula

A pinguecula is a yellow, triangular nodule found in the conjunctiva of the elderly and in people who work in exposed conditions. It affects the nasal side and later the temporal side. It does not spread to the cornea and no treatment is necessary unless it becomes inflamed, when steroid drops will reduce the condition. It can be removed for cosmetic reasons.

Concretions

Concretions are white deposits found in the conjunctiva. They are fairly common and are usually symptomless. Occasionally they are large enough to give a foreign-body sensation, when they can be removed under local anaesthetic (see p. 51). If bleeding occurs during this procedure, a pad and bandage should be applied.

Conjunctival cysts

Cysts can occur in the conjunctiva. If they cause symptoms, they are easily punctured under local anaesthetic (see p. 51). This can be a recurrent condition.

Chapter 8
The Cornea and Sclera

Introduction

The cornea and sclera comprise the outer, protective layer of the eyeball. The cornea forms the anterior one-sixth and the sclera the posterior five-sixths.

The cornea

The cornea is a transparent structure which fits into the surrounding sclera like a watchglass. It is convex, avascular and highly sensitive. The site where the cornea becomes continuous with the sclera is known as the corneal limbus.

Measurements

Vertical 10.6 mm; horizontal 11.5 mm; thickness 0.6 mm centrally and 1.0 mm peripherally.

The thinness of the cornea is significant and must be considered when removing corneal foreign bodies.

Five layers of the cornea

These are illustrated in Fig. 8.1

- Epithelium: there are five to six layers of epithelial cells, which are continuous with the conjunctival epithelium. The basement membrane is the innermost layer of the epithelium. The epithelium is the only layer of the cornea that regenerates following trauma.
- Bowman's membrane: a layer of connective tissue. Does not regenerate when damaged.
- Stroma: this comprises 90% of the cornea. It is composed of parallel connective tissue.
- Descemet's membrane: a layer of elastic fibres which regenerates when damaged.
- Endothelium: a single layer of endothelial cells which are metabolically active and their primary function is the control of stromal hydration. The endothelium elongates when damaged.

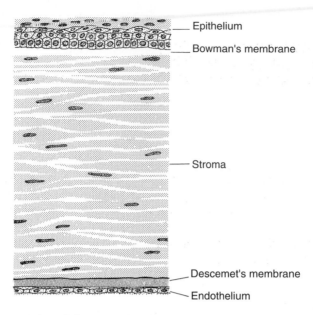

Epithelium
Bowman's membrane
Stroma
Descemet's membrane
Endothelium

Fig. 8.1 Transverse section of the cornea.

Functions of the cornea

Protection.

Refraction of light. The convex shape of the cornea allows most of the refraction of light rays within the eye to take place here, approximately 40 dioptres. The cornea must remain transparent to allow light rays to enter the eye and for sight to be clear.

Clarity is maintained by:

- Avascularity of the structure: no blood vessels to impede the transmission of light rays.
- Uniform structure of the stromal layer: the fibres lie in a parallel fashion; if they are pushed apart, for example by oedema, the structure becomes opaque and blurred vision results.
- Dehydration: the cornea is kept dehydrated by the endothelial layer. This is a sodium pump whereby sodium, and therefore water, is pumped out of the cornea to be replaced by potassium. Where this layer is damaged the pump ceases to work efficiently.

Blood supply

The blood supply and drainage is via the anterior ciliary artery and vein by limbal diffusion.

The cornea also receives some nourishment from aqueous and the tear film.

Nerve supply

The cornea is highly sensitive, receiving its nerve supply from the long ciliary nerve of the nasociliary nerve. This is the third branch of the ophthalmic division of the trigeminal nerve. The nerve endings lie under the epithelial layer.

The sclera

'Sclera' in Greek means 'hard'. The sclera is the 'white' of the eye, composed of dense, white, non-uniform collagen fibres. It is kept hydrated and is, therefore, opaque. The sclera extends from the cornea (the limbus) to the optic nerve.

It is 0.6–1.00 mm thick, although where the four recti muscles are inserted into it, it is only 0.3 mm thick. It has a protective function.

Areas of the sclera

There are four areas to note:

- Lamina cibrosa: a sieve-like structure where a few strands of scleral tissue pass behind the optic disc.
- Posterior aperture: lies around the optic nerve and is the area where the long and short ciliary vessels and nerves penetrate the sclera to travel forward in the eye to supply the choroid and ciliary body.
- Four middle apertures: situated at the 'equator' where the four vortex veins exit through the sclera.
- Anterior aperture: lies 4 mm posterior to the limbus where the anterior ciliary vessels puncture the sclera.

The limbus

The limbus is the transitional zone, 1.2 mm wide between the cornea, conjunctiva and sclera.

The episclera

The episclera is a fine elastic tissue covering the surface of the sclera. It has a rich blood supply from the long posterior ciliary arteries to nourish the sclera lying beneath it.

Scleral nerve supply

The ciliary nerve from the oculomotor nerve provides the nerve supply to the sclera.

Physiology of corneal symptoms

- Pain – due to many pain fibres being present in the cornea.
- Blurred or reduced vision – due to a lesion obstructing light rays entering and refracting at the cornea.
- Photophobia and watering – due to irritation of the corneal nerve endings.

Conditions of the cornea

Exposure keratitis

Exposure keratitis is an inflammation of the cornea resulting from drying of the cornea because the eyelids cannot protect it adequately. It is potentially a dangerous condition as, without treatment, it can lead to ulceration and perforation of the cornea.

The lids are unable to cover the cornea either because of proptosis of the eyeball or the inability of the lids to move over the eyeball. Once recognised, this condition must be treated promptly with measures being taken to protect the cornea. Bandage contact lenses can be used or a tarsorrhaphy performed with the use of eye ointment to form a protective layer.

Corneal ulcers

Corneal ulcers develop as a result of local necrosis of corneal tissue by bacteria, viruses, fungi or *Acanthamoeba*. The most common corneal ulcer is caused by bacteria such as *Staphylococcus, Pseudomonas* or *Streptococcus*. Bacterial invasion and infection can be as a result of corneal trauma, corneal foreign body, chronic blepharitis and contact lens wearing. Lid abnormalities such as entropion, trichiasis, and corneal exposure due to incomplete eyelid closure – such as Bell's palsy – may also lead to the development of corneal ulcer.

Signs and symptoms

- foreign body sensation
- aching
- pain
- red eye
- photophobia
- hypopyon in very severe cases
- lacrimation
- circumscribed opacity.

Patient's needs

- Relief of symptoms (severe pain, foreign body sensation, lacrimation, photophobia, reduced visual acuity).

- Antibiotic treatment to the eye.
- Address psychological needs.
- Address sleep deprivation due to frequency of drops.

Nursing action

- Prepare equipment and patient for corneal scrape.
- If the condition is severe and/or the patient is elderly, admit him to hospital.
- Give the prescribed antibiotics:
    - Intensive drops, e.g. G. Gentamicin and Cefuroxime (alternate) every half-hour for the first 24 hours. This means that the patient will be having drops instilled every 15 miutes. The frequency will be reduced according to the response.
    - Ointment, e.g. Oc. Chloramphenicol and Gentamicin at night at a later stage.
    - Subconjunctival antibiotics.
    - Oral antibiotics may be given especially if the ulcer is close to the limbus (Kanski, 2003).
    - If very severe, intravenous antibiotics may be given.
- Give analgesic drugs as prescribed.
- Instil topical mydriatics for associated uveitis.
- It is important to recognise signs of sleep deprivation – such as loss of appetite, depression, mood swings – and it is important that this is addressed. It is a good idea to nurse these patients in a side ward and make every effort to minimise the noise level. The room should be darkened and interruptions kept to a minimum. Patients should be offered warm drinks and a light diet. When patient is well enough, educate patient (and where appropriate relatives) in drop instillation technique in preparation for discharge home.
- It is also important to address any psychological needs of the patient. Good clear explanations at every stage of the management of the corneal ulcer will help to alleviate any anxiety and fear. Where appropriate, involvement of other agencies such as dietician, district nurses and social worker.
- If the patient is to be treated as an outpatient, instruct him in the instillation of drops and ointment as above. The frequency may be less, e.g. two-hourly. Ensure he has analgesics at home.
- Advise him to wear dark glasses for the photophobia but not to cover the eye with a pad. Explain that the pad could provide an environment in which the infection could thrive.
- Warn him that treatment may be prolonged, perhaps for several weeks until healing is complete.
- Topical steroids may be introduced once the ulcer begins to heal.
- Prepare the patient for botulinum injection to induce a ptosis which will cover the cornea.

Complications

- Scarring of the cornea occurs if the ulcer spreads beyond the epithelial layer.
- Uveitis with its own complications (see p. 123).
- Descemetocele formation: the elastic Descemet's membrane affords some protection against the spreading ulcer. The corneal layers above it have been destroyed and Descemet's membrane herniates through the ulcer. When this happens perforation may occur.
- Perforation of the cornea: this may be a dangerous situation as not only can sight be lost but the eye itself. If the infection is severe and has spread to the internal structures of the eye, the eye will need to be removed (see Chapter 15), as no useful vision will be saved and the patient will experience severe pain.

Corneal ulcers associated with viral infections

Adenovirus

These cause superficial punctate keratitis which is slightly raised dots on the cornea which show up when stained with G. fluorescein. These conditions have been discussed under viral conjunctivitis (see p. 92).

Herpes simplex

The herpes simplex virus causes an ulcer on the cornea which has a typical branching pattern and is called a 'dendritic ulcer'. It is usually unilateral.

Signs

- red eye
- dendritic ulcer (Fig. 8.2) seen on the cornea once stained with G. Fluorescein
- herpes simplex lesions may be evident around the eye
- cold sores may be present around the mouth and/or nose.

Patient's needs

- Relief of symptoms:
  - irritation
  - watering
  - photophobia
  - reduced vision.
- Pain may not be a symptom as the cornea may have become anaesthetised by the virus.
- Treatment for the infection.

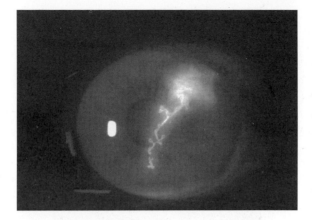

Fig. 8.2 Dendritic ulcer from herpes simplex virus.

Nursing action

- Take swabs for herpes simplex virus isolation.
- Instruct the patient on the treatment with antiviral agents: Oc. Acyclovir five times a day.
- Treatment is given for a week initially but may need to be continued for longer.
- Steroids are never used for herpes simplex infection because they increase the activity of the virus and the possibility of secondary infection. Perforation of the cornea has been caused by the use of steroids.
- Acyclovir cream can be applied to affected skin areas. Acyclovir cream for the skin must never be applied to the eye.

Complications

- Amoeboid or geographical ulcer: the dendritic ulcer spreads to take on the appearance of an amoeba or island.
- Disciform keratitis: the stromal layer becomes oedematous and there are folds in Descemet's membrane. The complaint occurs in patients who are immunosuppressed. It is usually a self-limiting condition lasting several weeks but may become chronic, in which case uveitis also occurs. A very low dose of steroids may then be required. G. Prednisolone sodium phosphate can then be produced in a weak solution such as 0.003%.
- Corneal scarring from repeated attacks of herpes simplex keratitis.
- If a corneal graft is performed, the herpes virus can attack the grafted cornea.

Herpes zoster ophthalmicus

This is caused by the herpes zoster virus attacking the ophthalmic division of the trigeminal nerve (Fig. 8.3). It therefore follows the path of the nerve

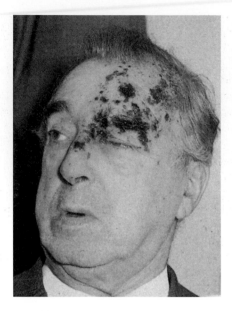

Fig. 8.3 Herpes zoster ophthalmicus.

over the forehead and into the eye. It usually affects the elderly and can be very debilitating. The disease starts with pain over the forehead and scalp on the affected side. A day or so later vesicles appear on the same area and may cover the upper lid. These then break down and weep serous fluid before drying up and forming scabs. The patient feels ill, anorexic and nauseated and may be pyrexial.

If the nasociliary nerve is affected, the cornea will be involved with white infiltrate and lesions may appear on the side of the nose. This is known as a positive Hutchinson's sign.

Patient's needs

- Relief of symptoms, especially pain.
- Admission to hospital if the condition is severe or if the patient is elderly and cannot manage at home.
- Institution of treatment.

Nursing action

- Ensure the patient understands the treatment.
- Skin lesions:
  - acyclovir cream can be applied twice a day to the vesicles
  - hydrocortisone cream can also be used.

- Corneal involvement:
  - antiviral agents, e.g. Oc. Acyclovir five times a day (Acyclovir can also be given orally)
  - antibiotics, e.g. G. Chloramphenicol four times a day to prevent a superimposed bacterial infection
  - steroids especially if there is stromal involvement, e.g. Betamethasone Sodium Phosphate drops four times a day, and a mydriatic, e.g. Homatropine 2% twice a day, to prevent or treat uveitis.
- Pain: oral analgesics such as paracetamol given regularly four-hourly. Stronger analgesics such as Mefenamic acid or Dextropropoxyphene may be necessary.
- Anti-inflammatory and anti-epileptic agents have been tried to treat the pain. Night sedation or an antidepressant at night may be required.
- Advise the patient that he will feel unwell and will require a light diet and plenty of fluids.
- Warn the patient that although the unaffected eyelid may swell in apparent sympathy, it will not be affected by the virus.

Complications

Fifty percent of patients develop ocular complications.

- Uveitis.
- Glaucoma.
- Cataract.
- Conjunctivitis.
- Keratitis.
- Permanent corneal scarring.
- Anaesthetic cornea due to the nasociliary nerve being damaged by the virus. The cornea is then exposed to damage because the corneal reflex is absent. Bandage contact lenses or protective arms on spectacles can be worn. This may resolve over months or years.
- More rarely, optic neuritis; scleritis; paralysis of the third, fourth and sixth cranial nerves.
- Partial ptosis due to scarring of lid from vesicles.
- Post-herpetic neuralgia is the most debilitating complication which can last intermittently for several years following the initial attack. It is difficult to treat and may require attendance at a pain clinic.

These complications can occur six to ten years after the initial attack.

Interstitial keratitis

Interstitial keratitis is due to congenital syphilis, manifesting itself when the patient is aged between 5 and 20 years. The disease can also occur as a result of other complications such as leprosy and tuberculosis. Tuberculosis is on the increase in this country (British Thoracic Society, 2004) as the number of immigrants and asylum seekers from countries with a high incidence of tuberculosis rises. Certain viruses such as measles virus, mumps virus can also cause a type of interstitial keratitis. There is involvement of the deep corneal layers and if left untreated, the entire cornea develops a ground-glass appearance. There is also invasion of new blood vessels from the limbus.

The patient complains of pain, watering eye, photophobia, and blepharospasm, and reduced vision. The eye is red and the cornea oedematous. Other signs of congenital syphilis may be present: saddle nose, deafness and notched incisor teeth.

There is no specific treatment. Any treatment given is aimed at preventing uveitis and the formation of posterior synechiae by giving mydriatics and steroid drops. Wearing dark glasses may help the photophobia. Corneal grafting may be necessary if corneal scarring becomes severe enough to obscure vision.

Bullous keratopathy

Bullous keratopathy is prolonged oedema of the cornea resulting in the epithelium being raised into large vesicles or bullae. It is a difficult condition to treat and the bullae may burst periodically causing intense irritating symptoms. It occurs following disturbance to the endothelium when aqueous is allowed to percolate into the stroma. This could be as a result of trauma, surgery (especially intra-ocular lens implants) or longstanding, poorly controlled glaucoma.

Hypertonic (5%) saline drops can be used to reduce the corneal oedema and improve vision (Kanski, 2003). Grafting may be necessary. Bandage contact lenses make the condition less painful and also flatten the bullae.

Corneal dystrophies

Corneal dystrophies can be categorised according to the corneal layer involved:

- epithelial/anterior Gogan's, map-dot, recurrent erosions, Reis-Bockler
- stromal granular, macular, lattice
- endothelial/posterior Fuch's.

These dystrophies cause increasing visual loss. Corneal grafting is the main form of treatment but the dystrophy can recur in the 'new' cornea. Recurrent erosions can be treated with the excimer laser.

Keratoconus

Keratoconus or conical cornea is due to a congenital weakness of the cornea, manifesting itself in the early teens. It can be associated with conditions such as eczema, learning disability or blindness as sufferers of these conditions tend to rub their eyes.

It is a bilateral condition, one eye usually being affected before the other. The central cornea becomes progressively thinner and more conical in shape (Fig. 8.4). The patient complains of blurred vision due to increasing astigmatism of the cornea.

Signs

- Munson's sign (see Fig. 8.4). When the patient looks downwards, the conical cornea causes an indentation of the lower lid margin.
- Distorted corneal reflection with Placido's Disc, a keratoscope, a pachometer or on corneal topography (Corbett et al., 1999).
- An irregular shadow on retinoscopy.
- Unclear view of fundus because of the corneal distortion.

Treatment

Initially the treatment will be with contact lenses to correct the astigmatism and protect the cornea. The astigmatism is too severe to be corrected by spectacles. As the conical shape progresses, an ordinary contact lens becomes useless. Grafting is performed, ideally before the cornea becomes too thin.

Complications

Acute hydrops of the cornea can occur as a result of rupture of Descemets's membrane usually due to eye rubbing by the patient. Over a period of time, acute hydrops usually clears spontaneously but often leaves scarring.

Keratoplasty – corneal graft

Keratoplasty needs to be performed when the cornea is so diseased that the patient's vision is lost (Fig. 8.5). It is performed for (in order of occurrence):

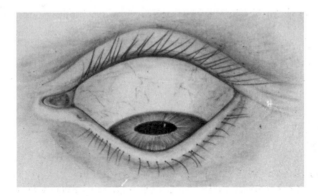

Fig. 8.4 Keratoconus. (Reproduced with permission from Miller, S. *Parson's Diseases of the Eye*, 16th edn, Churchill Livingstone.)

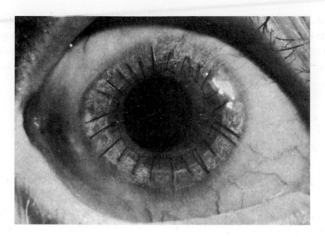

Fig. 8.5 Corneal graft.

(1)   keratoconus
(2)   bullous keratopathy
(3)   scarring/injury
(4)   corneal dystrophies
(5)   corneal ulcers
(6)   dendritic ulcers
(7)   failed previous grafts.

Eye donors

- Autogenous: rarely, a patient requiring a corneal graft has a fellow eye which is blind but with a healthy cornea which can be used for grafting.
- Live donor: an enucleated eye with a healthy cornea can be used for grafting onto another patient.
- Cadavers: most of the corneas used for grafting are obtained by this method. They must be removed within 12 hours of death and are stored in media. Organ culture medium permits storage for up to 30 days.

Donor corneas are not used from the following categories:

- corneal disease
- anterior segment surgery or disease
- HIV or hepatitis B positive and drug abuse
- death of unknown cause
- septicaemia
- leukaemia, Hodgkin's disease, lymphosarcoma.

A culture is taken from the eyes before removal to exclude any infection. Blood is taken to exclude hepatitis B and HIV. Both eyes are taken, including a part of the optic nerve. A suture is fed through the nerve and used to suspend the eye in a sterile jar to prevent the cornea becoming damaged. A prosthesis might be put in each socket or the eyelids are sutured together.

There are national eye donor banks in the UK in Bristol and Manchester, which store eyes waiting for recipients.

Human amniotic membrane transplantation

The first use of amniotic membrane transplantation (AMT) was in 1940 by De Rotth who used this technique in treating symblepharon. In 1946, Sorsby & Symons successfully treated patients with corneal burn following caustic burns. Since then, AMT has been used for persistent corneal epithelial defect (Lee & Tseng, 1997), leaking filtering blebs after glaucoma surgery (Budenz et al., 2000), Stevens-Johnson syndrome (Tsubota, 1996) and many other corneal diseases including systemic diseases which may cause ocular surface damage.

Human amniotic membrane is believed to be nonimmunogenic which makes it ideal in corneal graft in promoting non-rejection. AMT promotes epithelial healing, reduced inflammation, increased comfort, and decreased severity of vascularization.

Osteo-odonto-keraprosthesis (OOKP) surgery

Osteo-odonto-keraprosthesis technique is used in treating patients who are not suitable for conventional corneal graft surgery such as severely dry eyes or multiple corneal graft failure. The success of this type of surgery will depend on the lack of any previous ophthalmic history such as retinal disease, glaucoma and optic nerve involvement.

The surgery uses the patient's own tooth root and alveolar bone to act as vital support to an optical cylinder. The patient undergoes a vigorous pre-assessment check including a B-scan, assessment of the retina and optic nerve functioning and in some cases electroretinogram and visual evoked potential. The patient also has an oral assessment by the maxillo-facial surgeon and radiography where a decision is made as to which tooth to harvest. The canine tooth is usually harvested and in the absence of a suitable tooth, a relative's tooth may be used after suitable HLA match. The surgery is usually performed in two stages, which allow the growth of soft tissues around the osteo-odonto lamina and for the reconstruction of the ocular surface, by vascularisation. Potential complication could include buccal mucous ulceration in the early post-operative phase especially in smokers.

Eye tissue recipients

Patient's needs

- admission to hospital
- pre-and post-operative care.

Nursing action

- The nurse needs to ascertain that the patient understands that he will be receiving a donor cornea which is most likely to come from a cadaver. The use of the word 'graft' instead of 'transplant' may result in the patient being unaware of the true implications of this type of surgery. The nurse may want to involve the doctor or may discuss this with the patient on her own. Some patients may be distressed at the knowledge. Others having known for a while, may only face up to the fact at the time of surgery, while some may not have had the opportunity for discussion before. The nurse needs to be aware of those who require further discussion and talk it through with them.
- Admit the patient to the ward.
- Institute pre-operative care. The pupil may be constricted in penetrating keratoplasty to prevent damage to the lens during the operation unless a cataract is to be removed at the same time.
- Carry out post-operative care. At the first dressing ensure that the graft is in place, the sutures intact and that the anterior chamber is formed. Aqueous may have leaked through the suture line causing a flat anterior chamber. Instil antibiotic or antibiotic and steroid and mydriatic drops.
- Patients need to be advised about the signs of rejection: reduced vision, red eye, new vessel growth around the cornea and pain.
- Following corneal grafting, astigmatism may occur which will require correction by the wearing of spectacles or contact lenses.

Complications – short term

- Damage during the operation to the iris or lens.
- Aqueous leak from the graft which has lifted in one area. This will require resuturing.
- Infection requiring antibiotics.

Complications – long term

- Neovascularisation around the edge of the graft. No treatment is required unless vision is impaired. Beta rays can be used on the area to destroy the new blood vessels. Re-grafting may be necessary.
- Astigmatism caused by too tight sutures which may need adjusting. Topography can confirm this.
- Warping of donor graft caused by sutures that are too loose. This may require re-suturing.
- Rejection which will be treated with steroids. Compared with other transplant operations, keratoplasty does not present the same rejection problems as the cornea does not have a blood supply.

Corneal topography

Corneal topography uses computerised equipment to measure and calculate the curvature of the corneal surface points. The basic principle of corneal topography involves the projection of multiple light concentric rings onto the cornea. The reflected image is captured on a special camera and these images are analysed by computer software, with the results displayed in a variety of formats. These are known as topographic maps. Every map has a colour scale that assigns particular colour to certain keratometric dioptric range. Corneal topography is often used clinically for detecting and evaluating the severity of patients with keratoconus, postoperative healing patterns (excimer laser, photorefractive keratectomy – PRK), radial keratotomy and keratoplasty. The topographic diagnosis of keratoconus is often suggested by high central cornea power (normal cornea flattens progressively from the centre to the periphery), a disparity between the two corneas of a given patient and a large difference between the corneal apex and the periphery. However, long term contact lens wearer can inadvertently simulate early keratoconus.

Pachymetry

Pachometers measure the corneal thickness (normal corneal thicker in the periphery 1 mm reducing to 0.58 mm centrally) and are a good indicator for endothelial function. The endothelial cells can be photographed and counted – a procedure known as specular photomicroscopy. This involves a special mounted slit lamp like camera which allows the corneal endothelium to be visualised and photographed. The density of the endothelial cells can be counted as well as any endothelial cells deviating from normal (normal endothelial cells are hexagonal in shape). Conditions such as diabetes, anterior segment surgery, glaucoma and contact lens wearing can all contribute to endothelial dysfunction.

Management of corneal pain

Corneal pain is managed using topical non-steroidal anti-inflammatory agents.

The avascular cornea is one of the most sensitive tissues in the body, with the highest density of sensory neurones per mm just below the epithelium (Davies et al., 1984) four to five times greater than in the finger pads (Corbett et al., 1999). Any epithelial loss leads to the exposure of the sub-epithelial plexus nerve endings. Subsequently, the patient's main complaint will be one of pain. The management of corneal pain has often in the past been neglected and patients are frequently quite distressed as their pain can become almost intolerable. Their normal daily activities are often disrupted, including their sleep pattern. In addition to their pain, patients may also be complaining of a red eye, photophobia, foreign body or gritty sensation, lacrimation and a possible decrease in vision.

The most frequent cause of corneal pain, apart from surgery, is corneal abrasion. Traumatic corneal abrasion is one of the commonest causes of attendance in any emergency centre and these abrasions range from very small to large epithelial defect. Small abrasions usually heal without serious sequelae but larger and deeper corneal involvement can leave scar formation. Traumatic corneal abrasions can be as a result of any ocular injuries such as finger nails, twigs, foreign bodies, work-related injuries such as welding flash and chemical injuries. Other examples of possible causes of corneal abrasion include contact lens wearer, and epithelial disease such as dry eyes.

During the healing process of the corneal epithelium, the epithelial cells from the corneal limbus flatten and spread across the defect until it is covered completely. At the same time, new cells migrated from the basal layer of the epithelium.

The current management of severe corneal pain associated with a corneal abrasion is cycloplegics such as G. Homatropine 2% and advice to take oral analgesia. The use of topical non-steroidal anti-inflammatory such as Voltarol (diclofenac) or Acular (kerotolac) is not used routinely. A review of the ophthalmic literature in the use of non-steroidal anti-inflammatory in controlling corneal pain is well documented.

Jayamanne et al. (1997) report in their study that the use of topical Voltarol significantly reduced pain after traumatic corneal abrasion. Szerenyi et al. (1994) also studied the effect of Voltarol which significantly lowered corneal sensitivity in normal eyes and reduced discomfort, pain and inflammation following photo-refractive keratoplasty. Another study Brahma et al. (1996) reports on the use of Flurbiprofen as a topical analgesia for superficial corneal injuries and found that it provides more effective pain relief than traditional treatments for superficial corneal injuries. These patients also took less oral analgesia, had normal sleep pattern and took less time off work. McDonald (1998) examined the use of Acular for relief of corneal pain in 26 patients. It was found to be useful in controlling patients' pain. None of the studies showed any significant adverse effects from the use of topical non-steroidal anti-inflammatory. So far, no evidence exists in the medical literature that the use of non-steroidal anti-inflammatory interferes with the rate of corneal epithelial healing and this fact is well documented (McGarey et al., 1993; Hersch et al., 1990). This 'risk' is further reduced through limited dose and duration of use.

The routine prescription of a non-steroidal anti-inflammatory must be considered in any patients presenting with corneal pain following corneal abrasion on a verbal pain rating scale of four or more. Caution must be exercised in patients with a history of corneal ulcers, herpes virus infection, corneal dystrophies, post-operative corneal graft or recent ocular surgery within three months. In addition, any patients who are asthmatic or who have known allergies to any topical analgesia or non-steroidal anti-inflammatory should also proceed with caution.

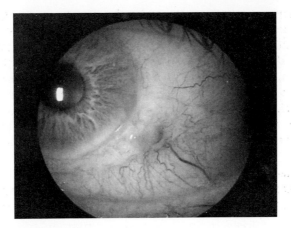

Fig. 8.6 Episcleritis.

Conditions affecting the sclera

Episcleritis

Episcleritis is inflammation of the episclera (Fig. 8.6). It may be unilateral or bilateral and can be associated with rheumatoid arthritis, gout and ulcerative colitis but the cause is often unknown.

There is a localised area of redness, usually triangular, with the apex pointing towards the limbus. There may or may not be a nodule present in the area of redness. The area is tender and, on examination, the conjunctiva moves freely over the enlarged episcleral blood vessels. Treatment is with non-steroidal anti-inflammatory such as Acular.

Scleritis

Scleritis is a rare condition affecting women more than men. In 50% of cases it is associated with connective tissue diseases, such as rheumatoid arthritis and ankylosing spondylitis. It can also be associated with uveitis, glaucoma and cataract. If it is anterior, the eye will be red, with tenderness over the affected area. If it is posterior, the eye will look white. Pain is the main feature and may be severe. Steroid drops will be used for anterior scleritis and systemic anti-inflammatory drugs such as ibuprofen for posterior scleritis.

Chapter 9
The Uveal Tract

Introduction

The uveal tract comprises the middle vascular pigmented layer of the eye. It is composed of three areas:

- the choroid, which forms the posterior five-sixths
- the ciliary body
- the iris.

These two latter structures (Fig. 9.1) together form the anterior one-sixth.

The choroid

The choroid lies between the sclera and retina and extends from the optic nerve forwards to the ora serrata where it joins the ciliary body. It is composed of four layers:

- the suprachoroid, containing pigment cells, elastic tissue and collagen
- the vascular layer, comprising large and small blood vessels with pigment cells contained in the stroma surrounding the vessels; the large vessels are mainly veins
- the choriocapillaries, comprising fenestrated capillary vessels
- Bruch's membrane, which is a barrier with fenestrations which allow nutrients through to the underlying retina; it is also a supportive membrane.

Function of the choroid

The function of the choroid is to provide nourishment to the outer layer of the underlying retina.

Blood supply

The blood supply and drainage is via the short posterior ciliary artery; and the choroidal and vortex veins.

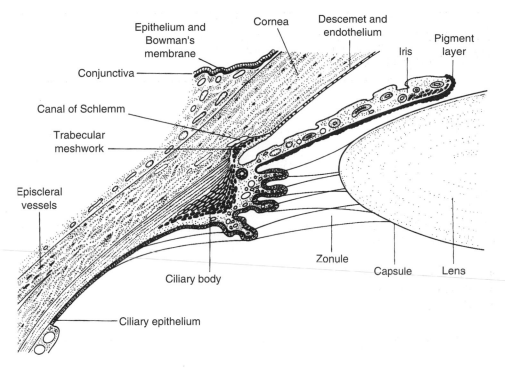

Fig. 9.1 Section through the iris and ciliary region.

Nerve supply

The posterior ciliary nerve from the oculomotor nerve provides the nerve supply to the choroid.

The ciliary body

The ciliary body is a triangular structure lying between the choroid and the iris, being 6 mm wide. It has three areas:

- The pars plana is the posterior aspect lying next to the ora serrata and is 4 mm wide.
- The pars plicata is the area which lies between the pars plana and the iris and is 2 mm wide. It contains 70–80 radiating strips, the ciliary processes. These processes are composed of vascular tissue, mainly veins and capillaries. They are 2 mm long and 0.5 mm wide. Their function is to produce and secrete aqueous which fills the posterior chamber and then flows through the pupil into the anterior chamber. The zonular fibres or suspensory ligaments, which hold the lens in place, originate in the valleys formed by the processes.

- The ciliary muscles lie in the anterior section of the ciliary body, underneath the sclera. The ciliary muscles are known as the muscles of accommodation. They contract and relax to change the shape of the lens so that light rays can be brought to a focus on the retina when looking at objects at varying distances. When the ciliary muscles contract, the zonules relax and decrease the tension on the lens capsule. The lens thus becomes more spherical and light rays can be focused on the retina for near vision. When the ciliary muscles relax, the zonules tighten and there is increased tension on the lens capsule. The lens thus becomes less spherical and light rays are focused on the retina for distance vision.

Blood supply

The blood supply to and drainage from the ciliary body is via:

- anterior ciliary arteries and veins
- long posterior ciliary arteries and veins
- vortex vein.

Nerve supply

The nerve supply is through the short ciliary nerve from the oculomotor nerve.

The iris

The iris is the coloured circular diaphragm situated behind the cornea and in front of the lens. It is attached at its periphery to the ciliary body. The pupil is the aperture in the middle of the iris. The iris forms the posterior wall of the anterior chamber and the anterior wall of the posterior chamber. There are two zones:

- the ciliary zone on the periphery
- the pupillary zone on the central aspect.

Three layers of the iris

- the endothelium
- the stroma containing connective tissue, pigment cells, blood vessels, nerves and muscles
- pigment epithelium which is an extension of the pigment epithelium of the retina (note that the epithelium of the iris is situated at the back of the structure).

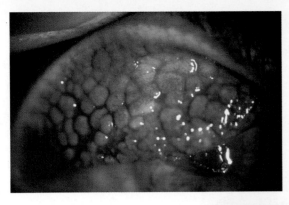

Plate 1 Cobblestone papillae.

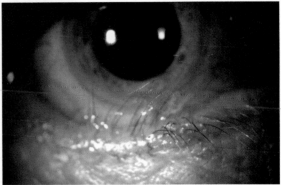

Plate 2 Trichasis with cicatricial pemphigoid.

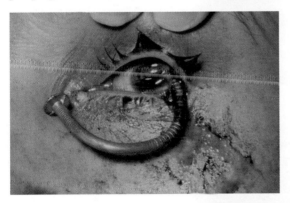

Plate 3 Penetrating injury.

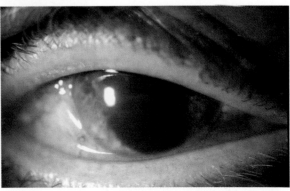

Plate 4 Hyphaema.

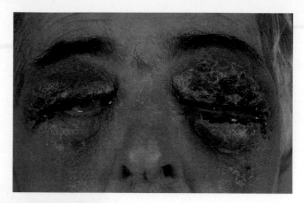

Plate 5 Bilateral orbital cellulitis.

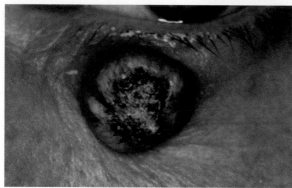

Plate 6 Rodent ulcer.

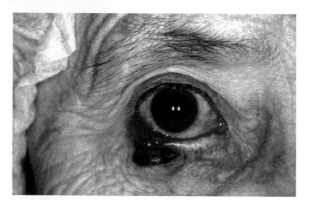

Plate 7 Basal cell carcinoma.

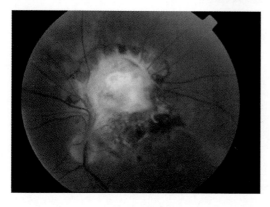

Plate 8 Toxoplasmosis.

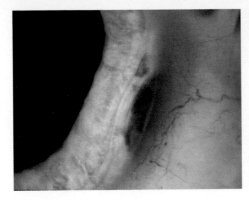

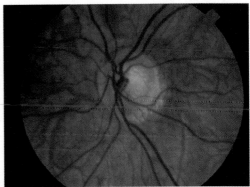

Plate 9 Iris melanoma.

Plate 10 Glaucomatous disc changes.

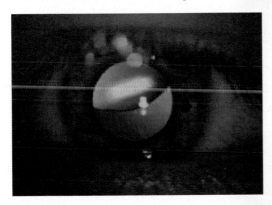

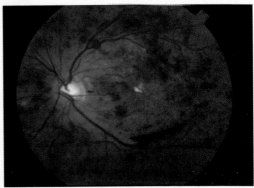

Plate 11 Subluxation of the lens.

Plate 12 Proliferative diabetic retinopathy.

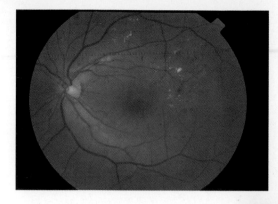

Plate 13 Background retinopathy.

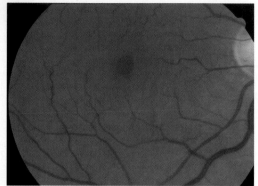

Plate 14 Macular hole.

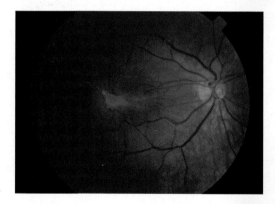

Plate 15 Epiretinal membrane.

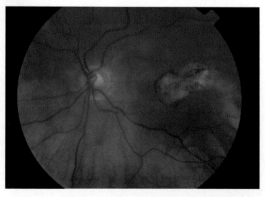

Plate 16 Macular degeneration.

Muscle of the iris

There are two muscles in the iris, whose actions are either to constrict or dilate the pupil:

- The sphincter muscle is a circular muscle lying around the pupillary zone. This muscle constricts the pupil. It is served by the short ciliary nerve of the oculomotor nerve.
- The dilator muscle is a radial muscle lying under the pigmented layer of the iris. As its name indicates it is the muscle that dilates the pupil and is supplied by the long ciliary nerve from the nasociliary nerve, the third branch of the ophthalmic division of the trigeminal nerve.

The sphincter muscle is more powerful than the dilator muscle, so if both muscles are equally affected by intra-ocular inflammation the pupil will tend to constrict. The sphincter muscle and the ciliary muscle both have their nerve supply from the oculomotor nerve, therefore drugs stimulating or paralysing this nerve will affect both dilation and accommodation.

Colour of the iris

The pigment melanin gives the colour to the iris. The colour depends on the amount of pigment laid down in the stroma after birth. This is genetically determined. The pigment in the pigment epithelium is present at birth and is consistent throughout life. This gives newborn babies light-coloured eyes. After a few days of life pigment begins to be laid down in the stroma and the baby's eyes become darker. The more melanin laid down, the darker the eyes become. All babies are therefore born with light-coloured eyes, despite what some doting parents may say. The amount of pigment produced in the stroma can vary during life, so that the colour of eyes can alter. Dark irises with dense pigment cause the pupil to take longer to dilate following instillation of mydriatics.

Blood supply

The arterial blood supply is via the long posterior ciliary arteries. The capillaries from these arteries anastomose with the anterior ciliary arteries to form the arterial circle of the iris. The venous drainage is through the anterior ciliary veins and vortex veins.

Conditions of the uveal tract

Anterior uveitis or iritis

Anterior uveitis or iritis is inflammation of the iris or iris and ciliary body (see Fig. 9.2). It is usually a recurring condition in which the cause is unknown in 70% of cases.

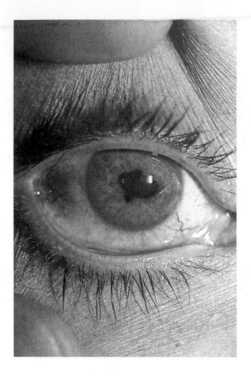

Fig. 9.2 Acute iritis.

Causes

Causes of anterior uveitis include:

- ankylosing spondylitis
- Still's disease or childhood arthritis
- seronegative rheumatoid disease
- ophthalmic surgery
- trauma – perforating injury, corneal foreign body
- corneal ulcer
- sarcoid
- tuberculosis
- syphilis
- ulcerative colitis and Crohn's disease
- rarely, neovascularisation from diabetes mellitus
- also rarely, heterochromic uveitis: patients with different coloured irises may develop this chronic, progressive condition in which the pigment of the affected eye is dislodged, with the iris becoming gradually paler.

Signs

- The visual acuity may be reduced.
- Ciliary limbal injection.

- Cornea is usually clear. Keratic precipitates may be present on the posterior surface of the cornea if the inflammation is severe. These are plaques of precipitates from the inflamed iris. In tuberculosis or sarcoid these are particularly marked and are called 'mutton fat' because of their appearance.
- The anterior chamber is of normal depth but 'flare and cells' may be seen in the beam of the slit lamp. Flares are as a result of exudative protein from the inflamed iris and cells are seen as leucocytes. Inflammatory cells may be sufficient in number to settle and form a hypopyon.
- The iris vessels may be dilated. A nodule may be present if the cause is tuberculosis.
- The intra-ocular pressure may be elevated.
- The pupil is small because the iris muscles are in spasm and the sphincter muscle is the stronger of the two iris muscles. The pupil will be irregular if posterior synaechiae has occurred when the posterior surface of the swollen iris adheres to the anterior surface of the lens.
- There may be cells in the vitreous
- Macular oedema may be present in severe anterior or intermediate uveitis

Patient's needs

- Relief of symptoms:
  - pain due to the spasm of the nerves of the iris
  - photophobia due to irritation of the nerves of the iris
  - watering eye again due to irritation of the nerves of the iris
  - reduced visual acuity due to the presence of flare and cells in the anterior chamber.
- Investigation of the cause in recurrent cases, and treatment, if applicable.
- Institution of treatment.

Nursing action

- Dilation of the pupil to prevent posterior synaechiae from forming or to break down any that have formed.
  - Instil prescribed mydriatic drops, often a 'cocktail' will be used, e.g. G. Phenylephrine Hydrochloride 10% and G. Cyclopentolate 1%. These may need to be repeated if synaechiae are present.
  - The application of heat by means of eyepads soaked in hot water and wrung out then placed over but not on closed lids will enhance the action of the mydriatics and cause the pupil to dilate quicker. The heat will also afford some pain relief. Do not apply the hot pads directly onto the closed eyelids.
  - A subconjunctival injection of mydriatics, e.g. Mydricaine may need to be given (see p. 43). This may be given in conjunction with steroids such as Betnesol.

- Ensure the patient understands the treatment to be instilled at home. This will be a:
  - mydriatic, e.g. G. Cyclopentolate 1% twice a day;
  - steroid, e.g. Prednisolone Forte 1% two-hourly or four times a day depending on severity.
- If investigations are to be carried out, ensure the patient understands where and when to attend for these. These tests will include: X-rays – skull, chest and joints to exclude sarcoid, tuberculosis, arthritis and ankylosing spondylitis; blood tests – haemoglobin, full blood count, erythrocyte sedimentation rate, serology and autoimmune profile.
- Ensure the patient knows when to return for follow-up treatment which will probably be in one or two days.

Often the management of patients with uveitis can be complex and time consuming and according to Jones (1998), the management of these patients must be optimised by early setting of targets for achievement, gaining patient's understanding and co-operation and by setting clear plans for management. Ophthalmic nurse practitioners have a large role to play in achieving these goals.

Complications

- Secondary glaucoma from three causes:
  - Posterior synaechiae, if not broken down, can cause a ring synaechiae when all of the pupillary zone of the iris is bound down to the anterior lens surface. The aqueous cannot flow through the pupil, so as the pressure builds up in the posterior chamber, the iris is pushed forward. This condition is known as iris bombe. Ring synaechiae can be divided surgically if mydriatics do not cause the pupil to dilate and thus break the synaechiae.
  - The peripheral anterior surface of the iris bombe adheres to the peripheral posterior surface of the cornea causing peripheral anterior synaechiae. These block the drainage angle.
  - Debris from the inflamed iris blocks the drainage angle.
- Cataract formation from impairment of the metabolism of the lens.
- Hypopyon of sterile pus.
- Cystoid macular oedema.

Choroiditis

Choroiditis is a condition manifesting itself as patches of inflammation on the choroid. On examination with an ophthalmoscope fluffy white patches can be seen through a hazy vitreous. When these patches heal, they leave pigmented areas of scar tissue.

Symptoms

The patient complains of reduced vision due to infiltrates in the vitreous and of an increased number of vitreous floaters. In 60% of cases, the cause is unknown. It can be caused by toxocara, toxoplasmosis (see Colour Plate 8) or syphilis. If the cause is known, this should be treated. A short course of high-dose steroids is also given.

Complications

- Cataract due to defective nourishment of the lens.
- Optic neuritis and secondary optic atrophy.
- Retinal changes and progressive degeneration, resulting in retinal atrophy – a decrease in the size of the visual field will be noted.
- Cystoid macular oedema (see p. 181).

Ophthalmic manifestations of HIV infection

Patients with HIV maybe presented with ocular manifestations involving the anterior or posterior segment of the eye. Due to recent advances in therapeutic agents for treating such infections, early diagnosis is important. All HIV patients should undergo an ophthalmological review so that prompt treatment can be instigated where appropriate. Anterior segment diseases of HIV includes Kaposi's sarcoma of the eyelids, conjunctiva and rarely the orbit. Herpes zoster ophthalmicus, herpes simplex virus and fungal infections can be associated with early clinical manifestations of HIV infection. Uveitis, Reiter's syndrome and syphilis are frequently seen in HIV patients. Posterior segment disease afflicting HIV sufferers involved the retina, choroid and optic nerve and are categorized into two: those associated with noninfectious causes and those infected with a variety of infectious disorders. Cytomegalovirus retinitis (CMV) is found in 25–40% of patients with HIV and is the most common retinal infection. Treatment for CMV included Ganciclovir or Foscarnet or a combination of both these agents.

Tumours

Benign naevi

These can be present in the uveal tract and must be observed carefully and regularly for malignant changes. They can be removed by laser. Melanomas are the variety of malignant tumour affecting the uveal tract. They are more common in the choroid but can occur in the iris and, more rarely, in the ciliary body where they carry a higher mortality.

Melanoma of the choroid

This can occur at any age but is more common over the age of 55 years. It usually occurs in the posterior pole and as it grows it pushes the retina forwards. A retinal detachment thus caused is often the first sign of a melanoma, so careful differential diagnoses must be made between a malignant and a simple retinal detachment. The edge of a malignant detachment is usually smoother than that of a simple detachment. Investigations include transillumination, colour fundus photography and ocular ultrasound. Treatment is with ruthenium or iodine plaques, proton beam radiotherapy, trans-scleral or trans-vitreal local resection or laser photocoagulation. The aim is to conserve the eye. Enucleation is reserved for patients who have visual loss, pain and poor cosmetic appearance, and those who are unable to cope with the thought of tumour spread or with prolonged treatment and follow-up. A length of optic nerve must also be removed with the whole eyeball. If the optic nerve is found to be involved on histological examination, radiotherapy should be given to the socket. The five-year mortality rate varies from 16% for small tumours less than 10 mm in diameter, to 53% for tumours larger than 15 mm (Damato, 1995). For nursing care following enucleation, see p. 220.

Melanoma of the iris

This is illustrated in Colour Plate 9. If a naevus in the iris is noted to be enlarging, local excision should be performed. The prognosis, providing treatment is prompt, is usually good.

Melanoma of the ciliary body

Ciliary body melanoma comprises of only 12% of uveal melanoma (Kanski, 2003). Due to the location of the ciliary body, small ciliary body melanomas are often quite difficult to locate and patients are often asymptomatic. Patients presenting with a large ciliary body melanoma may complain of a painless blurred vision due to secondary lens subluxation or astigmatism. Other secondary complications include hyphaema, cataract, retinal detachment and haemorrhage.

Chapter 10
Glaucoma

Introduction

There are numerous types of glaucoma and each has the potential to cause blindness. In the UK it accounts for 15% of blind registrations. A general characteristic of glaucoma is a rise in the intra-ocular pressure (IOP) that is sufficient to cause damage to the optic nerve head. IOP is determined by the balance between the rate of production and the rate of drainage of aqueous fluid. Normal intra-ocular pressure is 15–20 mmHg, but this measurement depends to some extent on which method is used to measure it. In addition, the thickness of the cornea can influence IOP readings. Thin corneas give rise to artificially low readings and thicker corneas may give rise to artificially high readings. For this reason, corneal pachymetry is performed.

Methods of measuring intra-ocular pressure

Digital

The patient looks downwards, closing the eye to be examined, and the nurse gently palpates the eyeball with the two index fingers to assess the degree of 'hardness'. This is not an accurate measurement but an eye with raised pressure will feel harder than one with normal pressure. It is a useful initial method of assessment, especially if none of the specialised equipment needed for measuring intra-ocular pressure is available, as in the GP's surgery.

Goldmann applanation tonometer

The tonometer head comprises a double prism. It is attached to a slit lamp. This is a contact method of determining the IOP, and the eye must be anaesthetised first with anaesthetic drops such as Proxymetacaine Hydrochloride 0.5%. Fluorescein sodium drops are also instilled to stain the tear film and allow the semicircles in the tonometer head (prism) to be viewed. The dial should be pre-set between 1 and 2. The cobalt blue light is used and the prism is placed against the cornea and the pressure measurement is read off a dial on the tonometer. The reading on the dial has to be multiplied by ten.

The tonometer should be calibrated on a daily basis to ensure accuracy.

Because of concerns about cross infection, disposable prism heads or prism sheaths should be used. Where non-disposable prisms are used, they must be properly disinfected between use.

Perkins' applanation tonometer

The Perkins' applanation tonometer is a hand-held tonometer, working on the principles of the Goldmann tonometer mentioned above. It is useful for patients who are unable to sit at a slit lamp, e.g. those who are in wheelchairs, who are bed-bound or unconscious. The method of use and normal pressure is the same as for the Goldmann tonometer.

Tonopen

Tonopens are small pen-like instruments that measure pressure in a similar fashion to the applanation method. This method is becoming increasingly popular as the operator does not have to have skill in the use of the slit lamp.

Non-contact tonometer

Non-contract tonometers, employed by optometrists, use a puff of air blown against the eye. The time required to flatten the cornea is converted into a figure to denote the intra-ocular pressure.

Schiotz tonometry

A contact method of measuring IOP that does not require a power source. This is rarely used in developed countries.

The anterior chamber

The anterior chamber is the area between the posterior surface of the cornea and the anterior surface of the iris. The angle of the anterior chamber may be examined using a gonioscope (see p. 134).

The posterior chamber

The posterior chamber is the area between the posterior surface of the iris and the anterior surface of the lens and suspensory ligaments. Both these chambers are filled with aqueous fluid.

Aqueous fluid

Aqueous is a clear fluid produced by the ciliary processes of the ciliary body (see p. 121). It flows from the ciliary body into the posterior chamber, through the pupil, into the anterior chamber, and drains through the anterior chamber angle at the rate of approximately 2 µl/minute.

Composition of aqueous

Aqueous is similar in constitution to plasma: 99% water and 1% nutrients, e.g. sodium, potassium, chloride, bicarbonate, glucose. Volume is approximately 125 μl.

Functions of aqueous

- to maintain intra-ocular pressure
- to provide a clear medium for refraction
- to provide nourishment to the lens; and to the posterior surface of the cornea.

The angle of the anterior chamber

The angle of the anterior chamber lies between the limbus (corneal–scleral junction) and the iris and it surrounds the circumference of the anterior chamber. It is composed of the trabecular meshwork and the canal of Schlemm (see Fig. 9.1). The trabecular meshwork is made up of fibrous connective tissue, perforated with oval holes (sieve like) and lined with endothelium, which is continuous with that of the posterior surface of the cornea. There are three distinct parts: the uveal meshwork, which is innermost extending from the iris root to Schwalbe's line; the middle section is the corneo-scleral meshwork – this is the largest section; the endothelial meshwork communicates directly with Schlemm's canal.

Aqueous drains via two routes: 90% through the meshwork from the anterior chamber into the canal of Schlemm. This is an oval-shaped channel lined with endothelium. Between 25 and 30 collector channels leave the canal of Schlemm and anastomose to form the intra-scleral plexus. From here the aqueous drains into the aqueous veins, the vortex veins and the inferior ophthalmic vein. The uveoscleral route accounts for the remaining 10% of aqueous drainage. Aqueous flows across the ciliary body to the suprachoroidal space, from here it enters the venous circulation.

Function of the angle

The angle is for the drainage of aqueous fluid from the eye into the venous circulation.

Blood supply

The blood supply to and drainage from the angle of the anterior chamber is via:

- anterior ciliary arteries
- aqueous veins.

Related disorders – glaucoma

Glaucoma is a group of conditions that can cause permanent sight loss. There is damage to the optic nerve head that may or may not be the result of a rise in the intra-ocular pressure. It is the damage to the optic nerve head that results in visual field loss (see Colour Plate 10).

The four types of glaucoma, each with a different aetiology, are:

- primary acute glaucoma (PAG)
- chronic open-angle glaucoma (COAG)
- secondary
- buphthalmos/childhood (ox-eye).

Primary acute glaucoma (acute closed-angle glaucoma)

Primary acute glaucoma (PAG) affects one in 1000 over the age of 40. The incidence increases with age and affects women four times more frequently than men. The condition can be divided into two types:

- primary pupil block
- primary irido-trabecular block.

Pupil block

Some 94% of PAG cases are of the pupil block type. The eye that is predisposed to this type has:

- a dome iris
- an iris that is characteristically bowed forward
- hypermetropia
- a shallow anterior chamber
- a narrow drainage angle
- a large anteriorly placed lens.

The pupil becomes blocked by the lens when the pupil is semi-dilated. The aqueous cannot flow through the pupil, resulting in a rise in pressure behind the iris. This causes the iris to be pushed forward (iris bombe) and the forward-placed iris blocks the drainage angle. Treatment for this involves the use of miotic drops such as Pilocarpine 2%, which brings the iris away from the angle and laser iridotomy which will allow the aqueous to pass into the anterior chamber, bypassing the blocked pupil. Beta-blockers such as Timoptol are used to reduce aqueous secretion in the affected eye and as a prophylactic measure in the other eye.

Note: Yag laser iridotomy is performed when the eye has responded to treatment, usually the next day and the fellow eye is also treated as a prophylactic measure.

Irido-trabecular block

Irido-trabecular block only occurs in 6% of PAG cases. In irido-trabecular block the eye typically has:

- a plateau iris
- emmetropia
- a deep anterior chamber
- deeply recessed angles.

Pupillary dilation leads to a progressive irido-trabecular blockage. Treatment is by the use of miotic drops to bring the iris away from the angle.

PAG usually presents unilaterally, but the fellow eye can also be affected, so it must receive prophylactic treatment.

PAG can be divided into five stages which may overlap but the overlap may not be orderly from one stage to the next:

- latent – asymptomatic
- intermittent or sub-acute
- acute
- chronic
- absolute – end stage.

Latent

As the patients are asymptomatic the condition is diagnosed either at a routine eye examination or when another eye condition is being investigated. These patients must be warned of the prodromal symptoms (see below) in case they progress to the next stage.

Intermittent or sub-acute

A rapid closure of parts of the angle (see Gonioscopy below) causes the pressure to rise. This results in certain prodromal symptoms and signs:

- headache
- eye pain
- blurred vision and haloes seen around lights due to corneal oedema
- nausea
- general malaise.

These prodromal symptoms and signs usually occur at night and improve by the morning when the miosed pupil during sleep has come away from the angle. Patients often think they have a migraine or 'sick headache'. An attack may develop into an acute attack or bypass this stage. As more of the angle becomes blocked with subsequent attacks, chronic closed-angle glaucoma develops. It is therefore important to diagnose and treat this stage early. Treatment is by laser iridotomy followed by intensive miotic drops.

Investigations

Provocative tests: Provocative tests are performed on patients with prodromal or latent symptoms to see if the intra-ocular pressure rises when the eye has been subjected to certain situations. Although rare, they are still in use in some centres.

Non-provocative tests – Gonioscopy: the depth of the patient's anterior chamber angle can be assessed by the use of a gonioscope. This is a large contact lens with either two or three mirrors placed at differing angles to each other (Fig. 10.1). This enables the angle of the anterior chamber to be viewed when used with the slit lamp. The patient's eye is anaesthetised with anaesthetic drops such as Proxymetacaine hydrochloride 0.5%. A lubricant such as Methylcellulose is applied to the surface of the lens that is placed against the cornea. This lubricates the lens and fills the space between the lens and the cornea. The degree to which the angle is open is graded using a grading system such as Shaffer. This system records the degree to which the angle is open on a scale from 0 to 4; 0 being closed and 4 being fully open. Grades 1 and 2 demonstrate that angle closure is probable/possible. The circumference of the angle usually has variable degrees of closure.

Acute glaucoma

This is an ophthalmic emergency as the acute raise in intra-ocular pressure can damage the optic nerve irreversibly.

Signs

- A sudden rise in intra-ocular pressure due either to pupil block or angle closure causes congestion and oedema of the structures involved.
- Lids may be red and swollen.
- Conjunctiva may show dusky red injection and may be chemosed.
- Hazy cornea.

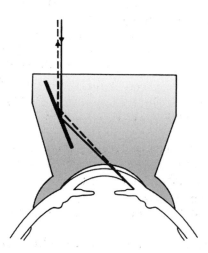

Fig. 10.1 Optical systems of Goldmann contact lens used in gonioscopy.

- Iris may appear 'muddy' and swollen with loss of its usual clear pattern.
- Pupil may be fixed, semi-dilated and oval in shape.
- Shallow anterior chamber.
- Raised intra-ocular pressure (can be as high as 70 mmHg or more).
- Rapidly reduced visual acuity.

Patient's needs

- Relief of symptoms: severe headache; pain in the eye; nausea; vomiting; abdominal pain; generally feeling unwell. These symptoms can sometimes be confused with other conditions such as acute abdomen and, with the dilated pupil, neurological conditions.
- Reassurance and explanation.
- Possible admission to hospital.
- Preparation for laser treatment.
- Instructions on discharge from hospital.

Nursing priorities

- Inform medical staff at once. Immediate treatment will bring relief of symptoms and prevent complications occurring.
- Prepare medication and commence instillation of drops as soon as possible after they have been prescribed.

Immediate nursing action

Test visual acuity, if patient is fit enough.

- Explain that treatment to the eye will relieve general symptoms.
- Lay the patient on a couch in a quiet, darkened area.
- Provide the patient with a vomit bowl and tissues.
- He may appreciate a cold compress on the forehead.
- Prepare Acetazolamide 500 mg to be given intravenously by the doctor to reduce the production of aqueous.
- Commence the instillation of G. Pilocarpine 4% four times per day to the affected eye once it has been prescribed. Intensive miotics are not effective in pulling away the iris from the angle as the sphincter muscle is usually ischaemic if the pressure is above 30 mmHg (Kanski, 2003).
- Commence G. Pilocarpine one to two times a day to unaffected eye.
- Commence a beta-blocker (e.g. Betagan – Levobunolol hydrochloride) to the affected eye.
- Commence steroid drops, e.g. Prednisolone acetate (Pred-forte) drops, to the affected eye as there is usually an associated inflammation.
- Give analgesics and/or anti-emetics if headache and nausea and vomiting continue despite treatment.
- Offer mouthwash if vomiting to freshen the mouth and breath (DoH, 2003).
- Prepare further treatment if necessary to reduce the intra-ocular pressure if initial treatment has failed to bring it down:

○   intravenous Mannitol 20%–200 ml given over one to two hours
  (i)   care for intravenous rate of flow and the site of the cannula, as
         leakage into the surrounding tissues causes phlebitis
  (ii)   assist the patient to the toilet or give a urinal or bedpan as Man-
         nitol has a diuretic effect.
○   Glycerol (1–5 mg/kg body weight) orally, in orange juice to disguise
    the taste. This in itself may induce nausea and vomiting.

The patient may resent the frequent attention he requires in the initial
stages of treatment of this condition and may just want to be left alone.
Handle the patient sympathetically and show understanding of his feelings.

Further nursing action

Prepare the patient for laser iridotomy to both eyes (prophylactically to the
fellow eye). Such preparation is restricted to explanation of the procedure
and ensuring that the patient has their pain assessed and appropriate analgesia provided before they attend for the laser treatment. If the patient is still
nauseous, anti-emetics should also be given as prescribed.

Chronic

Often referred to as 'creeping angle closure', this is when repeated attacks of
either intermittent or untreated acute episodes cause further adhesions of the
peripheral iris to the posterior surface of the cornea (peripheral anterior
synaechiae), thus closing the angle. The signs and symptoms are similar to
chronic open-angle glaucoma (see below).

Absolute

This is the end stage of primary acute, chronic and secondary (see below and
p. 144) glaucoma when treatment has failed. Cataracts are usually present
and occur due to the medical or surgical treatment rather than to the disease
process (Kuppens et al., 1995).
    Blind, painful eyes which occur at this stage are best treated by enucle-
ation (see Chapter 15). Alternatively, periodic retrobulbar or facial nerve
injections can be administered. Phthisis bulbi, or shrinkage of the eye, occurs
as it atrophies when enucleation is the most appropriate course of action.

Chronic open-angle glaucoma

Chronic open-angle glaucoma occurs in patients of either sex over the age of
45 years with symptoms usually occurring after the age of 65 if the disease
is undetected. This is not to be confused with the chronic form of primary
acute glaucoma. It has an insidious onset and is slowly progressive. The
patient does not usually notice symptoms until the disease has progressed

so far as to result in marked visual field loss. This is because it is the nasal visual field that is lost initially, the fellow eye compensates for the vision loss. It is a bilateral condition, with one eye often being involved earlier and more severely than the other. The patient usually first notices that he cannot see so well in his peripheral vision and has started knocking into things. He often thinks it is just old age or something a new pair of glasses will correct. Hence it is optometrists who often refer these patients to ophthalmologists.

Certain optometrists have received additional training in the diagnosis of chronic open-angle glaucoma. They have glaucoma suspects referred to them by fellow optometrists. The optometrist undertakes a thorough examination of the patient and only refers on to an ophthalmologist those people with glaucoma. This allows the patient reassured they do not have the disease and allows them to be discharged. It is thought that without such schemes as many as 20% of referrals to hospitals are false positives.

Cause

The cause of chronic glaucoma is not really understood, but there are several risk factors (Kanski, 2003):

- raised intra-ocular pressure
- family history
- history of migraine or vasospasm
- high myopia
- central retinal vein occlusion
- retinal detachment caused by a retinal hole
- Fuch's dystrophy
- increasing age
- diabetes mellitus
- raised systolic blood pressure.

There is also a higher incidence in the Afro-Caribbean population (Laske et al., 1994). The aqueous cannot drain away and the intra-ocular pressure rises. The optic nerve head is composed of millions of nerve fibres as they exit the eye. Where the central retinal artery and vein enter and exit through the middle of these fibres, this is referred to as the optic cup. In open-angle glaucoma the cup becomes larger as the nerve fibres atrophy, due to the pressure on them, producing loss of peripheral vision. Typically there is a loss in the nasal peripheral field at first, with progressive loss of the rest of the peripheral field (Fig. 10.2). Central vision is usually retained longer but will also be lost if treatment is not given or is unsuccessful. Sometimes patients experience loss of central vision before peripheral vision has been affected.

Chronic glaucoma affects 2% of the population and is familial in 10% of cases (Kanski, 2003). Anyone with immediate relatives with this disease should receive an ophthalmic check-up, which is free in the UK, every three to five years after the age of 40. Treatment can then be commenced as soon as signs occur, before symptoms are noted, so that sight can be saved.

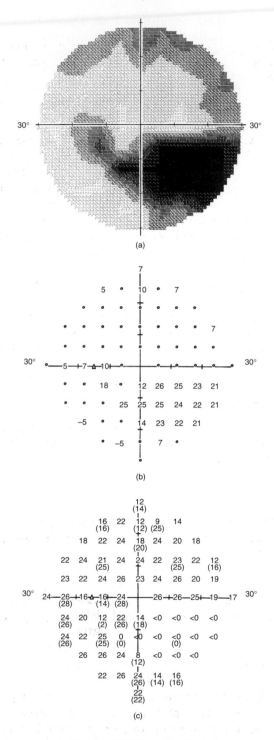

Fig. 10.2 Automated perimeter showing field loss which is shown as (a) a dark grey scale or (b) as high figures or (c) as low figures.

Investigations

Perimetry, posterior segment examination and applanation tonometry are carried out to diagnose and monitor the disease. Corneal pachymetry is also performed to determine the thickness of the cornea.

Perimetry

These tests are performed to assess the degree of peripheral and central visual loss (see p. 54). They are used to detect the disease and follow its progress. There are several different types of test but they all use the same principle. The patient, with one eye covered, stares at a white spot or light. Without moving his eye from this spot or light he indicates verbally or by pressing a buzzer as soon as he sees another spot or light entering his peripheral vision from any angle in the 360° circle. Most machines these days are computerised.

Posterior segment examination

Examination of the optic disc can be made using a slit lamp and hand held magnifying lenses such as 60 D; 78 D; 90 D, to assess the degree of cupping, state of the neuro-retinal rim and any changes to the retinal vasculature, e.g. bayoneting or flame haemorrhages.

Laser scanning tomography

This is a more sophisticated investigation of the optic disc which quantifies the areas of neural tissue at the optic disc by taking sections through the nerve head in a similar manner to a CT scan.

Tonometry

Measurement of the intra-ocular pressure is recorded (see p. 51). The pressure is not always markedly raised, especially early in the disease.

Gonioscopy

Gonioscopy will be carried out to assess the degree to which the angle is open (see p. 134). Patients may have narrow angles as well as chronic glaucoma.

Phasing

The patient normally attends as a day case to see if the intra-ocular pressure is raised at various times of the day. There is a normal diurnal pattern to IOP, with the pressure being higher in the mornings. The intra-ocular pressure is normally recorded every four to six hours, ideally by the same operator and with the same equipment.

HRT (Heidelberg retinal topograph)

3-dimensional topographic measurements of the optic disc and retina.

OCT (optical coherence tomography)

OCT uses laser to bring back information about the layers of the retina and also optic disc measurement. It is patient and user-friendly and dilation of the pupil is not essential.

Signs

- Cupped optic disc. The disc becomes oval vertically, and pale with the blood vessels being displaced nasally and the nerve fibre rim becoming narrower. A normal cup is 0.3; a glaucomatous cup is 0.5–0.8. (These values are expressed as ratios – the diameter of the cup is expressed as a fraction of the diameter of the disc giving a cup/disc ratio.)
- Loss of visual fields, typically peripheral field initially and central field later (Fig. 10.2).
- Raised intra-ocular pressure up to 25 mmHg.

Patient's needs

- An understanding of the condition, treatment and prognosis.
- Someone to listen and explain procedures.
- Advice about work/recreation/lifestyle changes.
- Guidance/help with mobility because of visual impairment.
- Information in a format that he can read and understand.
- Assistance with investigations, especially perimetry.
- Instruction in instillation of drops and taking of oral medication and the impact they have on the disease process.
- Preparation for laser treatment or surgery.

Nursing action

Guide/help patient while he is at the hospital. His degree of visual impairment will depend on the amount of glaucomatous damage. If he has peripheral field loss, he will tend to knock into furniture, doors, etc, and will need to be escorted to the varying departments during his visit. McBride (2000 and 2002) found that hospitals were not meeting the needs of people with visual impairment. Patients need people to respect them as human beings and not just another case. Nurses should be pro-active in ensuring that the environment is conducive to the needs of people with visual impairment.

Assist the patient with or perform perimetry. These tests require concentration on the part of the patient. As many patients are elderly this is not easy to maintain and therefore the patient needs encouragement and assistance during these tests.

Provide the patient with information on his treatment and treatment options which will be either:

- Medical – it is not wise to employ more than two topical medications as changes to the conjunctiva which may occur after three years' use may compromise the success of a trabeculectomy (Broadway et al., 1994). Most frequently, the choice will be mono therapy initially.
- Laser – effective in short-term control (Migdal, 1995).
- Surgical – surgery is now being performed earlier in the disease than in the past (Migdal, 1994). When performed early in the disease the intra-ocular pressure is well controlled (Migdal, 1995). It is important to emphasise that lost sight cannot be restored and that the aim of treatment is to preserve what sight is remaining.

Medical treatment

The model for the management and treatment of people with open-angle glaucoma is increasingly a shared responsibility. Nurses and optometrists have expanded their roles to include managing caseloads of patients with stable glaucoma. Protocols and guidelines following risk assessment support such roles.

As compliance can be a particular problem in this chronic condition (Patel & Speath, 1995) there is a need to emphasise the importance of instilling the drops in order to control the IOP, with a view to preventing further visual field loss. Following clinical examination and interpretation of results, discussion with the patient should be about explaining findings, ensuring they have an understanding of what has been said. Answer any queries the patient may have. A target IOP will be set, usually 30% reduction from the baseline measurement (EGS, 2003). When setting the target pressure factors relating to the patient's quality of life should be taken into account such as their level of anxiety relative to the chronic nature of the condition, current level of vision loss, cost, inconvenience and side effects of treatment.

Instruct the patient about his drops and any other medication; they need to be aware of the effects and side effects. The following medications may be instigated:

- Prostaglandin analogues, e.g. Latanaprost 0.005% or Travoprost 0.004% nocte.
- Beta-blocker, e.g. Timolol maleate (Timoptol) twice a day or Betaxolol 0.25% twice a day.
- Miotics, e.g. Pilocarpine 1%–4% four times a day.
- Acetazolamide tablets 250–500 mg four times a day or slow-release twice a day.
  With drop instillation, there is a need to prevent systemic absorption. This can be achieved by asking the patient to close their eye gently after instilling the drop and count slowly to 60 before they open it again.
- Combined topical preparations, e.g. Cosopt (dorzolomide 2% and timolol 0.5%) or Xalacom (latanoprost 0.005% and timolol 0.5%).

Where topical medication proves to be ineffective, consideration should be given to changing the medication before adding additional medication. Medication may be added where there is some response to treatment but the target IOP has not been achieved. (MREH, 2004).

Laser treatment

Prepare the patient for laser (see p. 48) trabeculoplasty. This procedure involves bombarding the trabecular meshwork with the laser. It is thought that scarring of the tissue stretches the meshwork and opens it up.

Surgical treatment

Admit patient to the day unit or ward.

- Prepare patient for operation, which is usually performed under a local anaesthetic unless there are indications for general anaesthetic.

    Trabeculectomy is the commonest type of drainage operation performed. This operation involves making a scleral flap and removing a strip of trabecular meshwork below this flap. The scleral flap is sutured back into place, but as this does not heal properly, it causes a fistula through which the aqueous can drain into the scleral vessels. The bulge over the scleral flap, lying under the conjunctiva, is called a 'bleb'.

- Give post-operative care:
    - Eye dressing:
        (i)   Remove and discard the cartella shield.
        (ii)   A bleb should be noted under the conjunctiva.
        (iii) The anterior chamber will be shallow but should not be flat. If it is flat, the bleb is probably draining too much aqueous. A firm pad and bandage should be applied to seal the bleb. The medical staff should be notified.
    - Instillation of drops:
        (i)   antibiotic
        (ii)   steroid
        (iii) mydriatic.
- Discharge of patient. If he is receiving antagonistic drops to each eye he must be warned of the danger of a mix-up. The operated eye may be receiving a mydriatic and the unoperated eye a miotic as treatment for chronic glaucoma. He may need to be reminded to continue to take the medication to the unoperated eye.

Complications of trabeculectomy

Early

- over-drainage
- under-drainage
- hyphaema
- aqueous misdirection into posterior segment of eye.

Late

- Subconjunctival fibrosis: patients who have had long-term medical treatment prior to their surgery are more prone to fibrosis (Broadway, 1994). Cytotoxic agents, such as 5-fluorouracil or mitomycin, given at the time of surgery or a few days post-operatively, can prevent this occurring (Kanski, 2003). Care must be taken when handling cytotoxic agents. Wear protective gloves, goggles, facemask and apron when drawing it up. Ensure correct disposal of used syringes, needles and other equipment used in an appropriately labelled container.
- Cataract formation due to surgical intervention.
- Infection as the bleb/fistula is only covered by conjunctiva.

Ocular hypertension

Intra-ocular pressure is higher than normal, over 21 mmHg on more than one occasion, and yet there is no damage to the optic disc and no visual field loss. The condition may never progress to open-angle glaucoma.

Risk factors

- age – increasing age
- race – Afro-Caribbeans and mixed race
- gender – affects women more than men
- type II diabetes
- systemic hypertension
- family history of glaucoma
- corticosteroid treatments.

Normal tension glaucoma

This is sometimes referred to as low-tension glaucoma.

Risk factors

Age, affecting the elderly and women more than men. It is seen more often in Japan than in Europe or the USA.

Clinical presentation other than IOP is similar to open angle glaucoma and treatment is also the same. Blood pressure is monitored and dips in systemic blood pressure, especially at night, should be noted. Any anti-hypertensive medication should be avoided at night.

Secondary glaucoma

Secondary glaucoma can be due to any of the following causes:

- Conditions of the lens:
  - Dislocation (see p. 159). The dislocated lens falls into the drainage angle or into the posterior chamber blocking the pupil.

○ Cataract formation (see p. 149).
    (i)   The enlarged lens pushes forwards, blocking the pupil or angle. This is called intumescence of the lens.
    (ii) Lens material oozes out through the lens capsule clogging the angle. This is called phacolytic glaucoma.

- Conditions of the uveal tract:
  ○ Uveitis (see p. 123).
      (i)   Debris from the inflammation of the uveal tract may clog the drainage angle.
      (ii) Pupil block caused by posterior synaechiae.
      (iii) Permanent peripheral anterior synaechiae may develop from repeated attacks of uveitis.
  ○ Tumours (see p. 127). Melanomas in the uveal tract cause raised intra-ocular pressure by volume replacement, encroachment on the angle or by blocking the vortex veins.

- Trauma:
  ○ Haemorrhage (hyphaema; see p. 215) into the anterior chamber. The blood in the anterior chamber clots in the angle effectively obstructing aqueous outflow.
  ○ Angle recession.
  ○ Corneal or limbal laceration (see p. 213). The anterior chamber is flattened and the angle closed by adherence of the anterior surface of the iris onto the posterior surface of the cornea.

- Post-operative causes:
  ○ Flat anterior chamber: following intra-ocular surgery, aqueous may escape through the wound, causing a flat anterior chamber. If this persists, permanent anterior and posterior synaechiae may develop.
  ○ Post-operative hyphaema: blood clotting in the angle blocks the drainage channels.

- Rubeosis iridis: in diabetes mellitus and following occlusion of the central retinal vein, small blood vessels grow into the anterior surface of the iris (neovascularisation) and into the angle of the anterior chamber where they may block the drainage channels (thrombotic glaucoma). The new vessels may also cause a spontaneous hyphaema.

- Steroids: it is not clearly understood why long-term treatment with topical steroids cause a rise in intra-ocular pressure. Care must be taken in the use of topical steroids in patients with a family history of chronic glaucoma. Regular checks of intra-ocular pressure in these patients and in long-term users of topical, and in some cases, systemic, steroids must be undertaken.

- Thyroid eye disease: infiltration of the orbital fat and extra-ocular muscles pushes the globe forwards, causing pressure on the globe with a subsequent increase in intra-ocular pressure.

Patient's needs

These are similar to those of primary acute glaucoma. A careful history must be taken because of the similarity in presenting signs and symptoms to primary acute glaucoma, and the other eye must be examined for depth of the anterior chamber.

Nursing action

The cause of the secondary glaucoma, once diagnosed, is treated first. Therefore the nursing action will be that of the cause.

The intra-ocular pressure is reduced by medical treatment initially. Surgical intervention may be required if medical treatment fails to keep the intra-ocular pressure within normal limits. Nursing action will therefore be instruction of the patient on instillation of drops and taking medication, and administration of pre- and post-operative care when surgery is performed.

Buphthalmos/childhood glaucoma (ox-eye)

Buphthalmos is a rare congenital condition affecting one in 10 000 births and resulting in increased intra-ocular pressure caused by a defect or blockage of the drainage angle by an embryonic membrane. Occasionally the canal of Schlemm is absent. Forty percent have raised intra-ocular pressures in utero, 50% manifest in the first year of life and 10% manifest between the first and third year of life.

It is usually a bilateral condition, boys being more commonly affected than girls.

Signs

- Large bulging eyes (Fig. 10.3). In childhood the sclera is more elastic than in the adult eye and the ever-increasing intra-ocular pressure stretches the sclera. It becomes thinned and appears bluish due to the pigment of the uveal tract showing through. The cornea also stretches. The enlargement of these two structures gives the child's eye the appearance of an ox-eye.
- Deep anterior chamber. The lens is pushed backwards by the increased pressure, thus forming a deep anterior chamber.

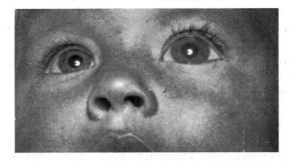

Fig. 10.3 Buphthalmos.

- Large cornea. As the cornea is stretched, its diameter increases from a normal 9.0–11.5 mm to 12–14 mm. Tears may appear in Descemet's membrane.
- Deep cupping of the optic disc due to the raised intra-ocular pressure.
- The intra-ocular pressure will be between 25 mmHg and 45 mmHg.

Patient's needs

- Relief of symptoms:
  ○ lacrimation – child always appears to have running eyes and nose
  ○ photophobia – child often puts his arm over his eyes to shield them from the light
  ○ general irritability.
- Admission to hospital.
- General care of a child in hospital.

Nursing action

- Admit the child to the paediatric ward.
- Give an explanation and reassurance to the parents or guardians. Involve them in as much of the child's care as possible.
- Prepare the patient for examination under anaesthetic. The following investigations are carried out:
  ○ measurement of intra-ocular pressure
  ○ gonioscopy
  ○ ophthalmoscopy of optic disc
  ○ measurement of corneal diameter.

These investigations are performed initially to diagnose the disease and thereafter at periodic intervals to assess success of treatment or progress of the disease.

- Give post-anaesthetic care following examination under anaesthesia.
- Administer pre-operative care if surgery is to be performed:
  ○ A goniotomy will be performed to open up the drainage channels by sweeping a goniotomy knife around the whole of the anterior chamber angle.
  ○ A drainage operation, such as a trabeculectomy, will be performed where the canal of Schlemm is absent or if the goniotomy fails to keep the intra-ocular pressure within normal limits.
- Give post-operative care:
  ○ monitor for pain and give prescribed analgesia
  ○ instillation of antibiotic and/or steroid drops – a mydriatic may be used
  ○ observation of the 'bleb' and depth of anterior chamber following trabeculectomy (see p. 142).

If the glaucoma is unilateral, amblyopia must be prevented in that eye (see p. 188). Patching of the unaffected eye will be instituted to encourage the child to use the glaucomatous eye.

Prognosis

The prognosis depends on when the disease became manifest (see above). The earlier the disease is present, the worse the prognosis, and visual impairment may be severe.

Complications

- Corneal/scleral perforation due to the thinning of those structures. Perforation may occur with the least trauma.
- Exposure keratitis due to the lids being unable to lubricate the enlarged cornea adequately.

A bandage contact lens can be used to prevent and treat both these conditions.

Juvenile glaucoma

Juvenile glaucoma is associated with neurofibromatosis, Sturge-Weber syndrome, rubella and aniridia. It presents later than buphthalmos and behaves like chronic open-angle glaucoma. Hence care of the patient is similar.

Chapter 11
The Crystalline Lens

Introduction

Structure of the lens

The lens is a biconvex, transparent, avascular structure with no nerve supply (Fig. 11.1). It measures 9 mm by 4 mm in diameter. The lens lies behind the iris and in front of the vitreous. It is supported by the zonules or suspensory ligaments, which attach it to the ciliary processes.

The lens has an elastic capsule, which enables it to change shape during accommodation (see p. 121). This capsule is semipermeable to water and electrolytes. The lens receives its nourishment from the aqueous humour.

The anterior surface has a single layer of epithelial cells. The anterior pole is less convex than the posterior pole.

The cortex of the lens is composed of a gelatinous substance and lamella fibres, which are arranged in layers, like an onion and originate from the anterior epithelial layer. These fibres are continually being produced so that the lens enlarges slowly throughout life, compressing towards the centre. Where the lamella fibres meet end-to-end, suture lines are formed. In the nucleus these are Y-shaped and when viewed with the slit lamp, can be seen to be erect anteriorly, i.e. Y, and inverted posteriorly, i.e. λ.

The nucleus is composed of sclerosed lens fibres. These are old cortical fibres that cannot be cast off and are therefore massed together in the centre as the nucleus. The nucleus grows in size and is harder than the cortex.

Composition of the lens

The lens is 65% water and 35% protein. In addition, there are trace minerals, the most important being sodium, potassium and calcium.

Function of the crystalline lens

The function of the lens is to focus light rays on the retina by 'accommodation' (see p. 121). The lens has a power of approximately 21 diopters (21 D). After the age of 45 years, the lens has become so solid that it gradually loses its ability to change shape. This means that the lens cannot accommodate for near vision, a condition called presbyopia. Spectacles are therefore needed

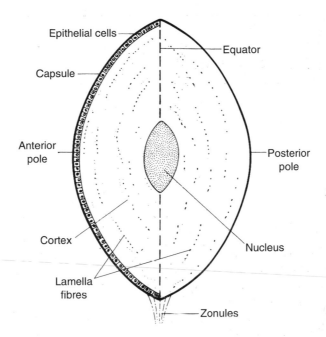

Fig. 11.1 Cross-section of lens structure. (Reproduced with permission from *Ophthalmic Nursing*, Smith & Nachazel (1980), published by Little, Brown and Company.)

for reading and close work. The presbyopia slowly progresses until about the age of 70 years, those affected requiring increasingly stronger lenses for reading and fine work.

Cataract

A cataract is an opacity of the crystalline lens. The lens is a delicate structure and any insult on it causes absorption of water, resulting in the lens becoming opaque.

Cataracts can be defined according to their type, location and degree.

The types of cataract

- congenital
- age related
- familial
- traumatic
- toxic
- secondary to existing eye disease
- associated with systemic disease.

Location of the opacity

Cataracts can occur in different parts of the lens:

- anterior pole cataract
- posterior pole cataract
- nuclear cataract
- cortical cataract
- lamellar cataract.

Degrees of cataract

- Immature cataract – part of the lens is opaque.
- Mature cataract – the whole lens is opaque and may be swollen (intumescent) (see Fig. 11.2).
- Hypermature cataract – the lens becomes dehydrated because water has escaped from the lens, leaving an opaque lens and wrinkled capsule.
- Phacolytic lens – lens matter leaks out causing uveitis and secondary glaucoma. Cataracts should be extracted before this situation arises.

The mature and hypermature cataracts can be viewed through the pupil. An immature cataract can be seen when viewed with a slit lamp.

Congenital cataract

Causes

- Rubella or malnutrition in the first trimester of pregnancy results in a lamellar cataract in the baby.
- Abnormal development of the eye in the fetus causes pressure on the anterior pole, resulting in an anterior pole cataract.

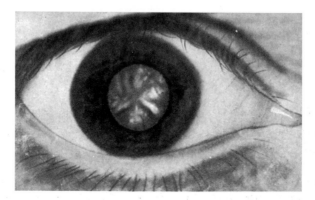

Fig. 11.2 Mature cataract.

- A tag of hyaloid membrane remaining from fetal life can result in a posterior pole cataract (the hyaloid artery runs from the retina to the lens during fetal life).
- Metabolic disturbance such as galactosaemia results in a nuclear cataract.

Signs of a cataract in a baby or child

- A white pupil may be noted by the parents or health visitor. It may be unilateral or bilateral. The cause of the white pupil must be diagnosed to differentiate it from the more serious condition retinoblastoma (see p. 177).
- The parents may notice that the child does not see well. They may also notice changes in the child's behaviour such as loss of concentration as they cannot follow word, pictures, etc., inability to catch a ball because of loss of depth perception.
- A squint will indicate that there is a lesion in the visual pathway preventing the sight from developing. The cause again must be differentiated from a retinoblastoma.
- It is important that cataracts are removed as soon as possible to prevent amblyopia occurring (see p. 188). This is especially important if the cataracts are bilateral and dense, when extraction should be carried out before the baby is two months old.
- The rule of thumb is that if the fundus can be seen, then light must be reaching the retina. Amblyopia (see p. 188) will therefore not develop. Removal of the lens will itself cause amblyopia as the light rays are not directed onto the retina by the lens. Compliance with aphakic correction (see p. 156) is therefore very important in these children.

Familial cataract

Familial cataracts can occur, but they are rare, affecting the 30–40 year age group.

Age related cataract

Age related cataracts occur in patients over the age of 60 years. They result from sclerosis of the lens due to a degenerative process. The rate of progression varies. It is usually a bilateral condition, one eye being affected before the other.

The cataract is either nuclear or cortical.

A nuclear cataract affects the central lens and takes on a brown colour. In this instance the patient sees better in dim light when the pupil is dilated and the light rays can enter the eye around the central opacity. Mydriatics can be given to dilate the pupil and give some vision around the cataract.

A cortical cataract affects the periphery of the lens and looks white. This type of cataract can produce a uni-ocular diplopia as the opacity splits the light rays. Vision is usually better in bright light when the pupil constricts and so reduces the peripheral distortion.

Traumatic cataract – see p. 217

Toxic cataract

Toxic substances can affect the metabolism of the lens and cause opacity formation. Radiation and drugs such as topical steroids have this effect.

Cataracts secondary to existing eye diseases

Glaucoma, retinitis pigmentosa, retinal detachments, retinopathies, choroiditis and uveitis upset the metabolism of the lens, causing cataract formation. The opacities form in the posterior sub capsular area, eventually involving the entire lens.

Cataracts associated with systemic disease

Some systemic diseases cause an upset in the metabolism of the lens, causing, in the main, posterior sub capsular opacities.

Diabetes mellitus, Type 1 and Type 2: the increased glucose level in the aqueous humour is taken up by the lens disturbing its metabolism. Cataracts can occur with rapid onset in juvenile diabetics, the lens becoming completely opaque within several weeks. In older diabetic patients the opacities are nuclear, posterior sub-capsular or cortical in nature and take longer to develop.

Hypoparathyroidism: cataract formation from this cause is usually seen after the removal of the parathyroid glands during thyroid gland removal. It can be idiopathic. Low calcium levels disturb the lens metabolism.

Atopic disease: dermatological conditions such as eczema and scleroderma can, when severe and widespread, cause cataract formation.

Effects on vision of a cataract

Patients with cataracts complain of gradually fading vision, often complaining that their vision is 'misty'. Other visual disturbances include distortion of images, changes in colour vision. Depending on the site of the cataract, as has been mentioned above, they may be able to see better in dim or bright conditions. Some complain of dazzling bright lights due to irregular refraction of rays through the opacities in the lens. Some patients experience monocular diplopia. Posterior capsular opacities cause difficulty in near vision, leaving distance vision unaffected.

Patient's needs

The patient's needs are many and varied but include information on the following:

- knowledge of the condition
- how the cataract will be treated and whether they will have an artificial lens implanted
- type of anaesthetic
- informed consent to the surgery
- when they can have the surgery
- how long they will be at the hospital or treatment centre
- how their vision will be after the operation and how long before they can get new glasses
- how to manage their post-operative eye drops
- how to clean their eye
- wearing the cartella shield at night time (usually at night for one or two weeks only)
- recognising and managing post-operative complications
- resuming normal activities
- written information/advice sheets
- detail of any follow up appointment
- how soon the other eye can be operated on (if needed).

Cataract extraction is normally performed as a day case unless there are factors that require inpatient admission. The waiting times for cataract surgery are much shorter, some centres having no waiting list at all.

Pre-assessment

Many centres now have cataract pathway management documents to guide the process from first visit to discharge. These may be accessed electronically or as hard copy. They are designed to streamline care from the multidisciplinary team. The patient may be seen by optometrists and nurses for the pre-operative and post-operative management phase of care, only seeing the doctor for the surgical procedure itself.

Special needs should be identified at or before the pre-assessment visit – such as the need for an interpreter, whether transport is needed, etc.

Pre-operative investigations

Keratometry (see p. 53).
Biometry (see p. 53).

'B' Scan

The 'B' Scan is an ultrasound scan used before cataract extractions. It gives a three-dimensional picture of the eye, showing up any abnormality in the media, such as a retinal detachment or tumour. This examination is necessary because the ophthalmologist is unable to examine the fundus through an opaque lens. If a tumour or retinal detachment were noted, the lens extraction might not take place, as no improvement in vision would occur.

Visual potential may need to be tested for because, for example, a patient may not have good post-operative visual acuity due to undiagnosed, age-related macular degeneration (see p. 179). OCT (see p. 140) is an example of a diagnostic tool.

Pre- and post-operative care

Nursing action

- Prepare the patient for a general or local anaesthetic. Probably the most frequently used local anaesthetic method now is Sub-Tenon's as it has fewer complications/risks than more traditional methods. Some ophthalmic surgeons advocate the use of topical local anaesthetic agents. The pupil will be dilated before surgery so that the surgeon can see and access the cataract during surgery.
- Give post-operative care.
- Eye care:
  - On examination with a good pen-torch or slit lamp, the conjunctiva will be mildly injected:
    - (i)   the cornea should be clear
    - (ii)   the anterior chamber should be deep and quiet
    - (iii) the pupil should be central – it may still be dilated from the effects of the pre-operative mydriatics and slightly eccentric initially.
  - If a posterior chamber intra-ocular lens is in situ, its reflection may be noted through the pupil.
  - An antibiotic and steroid drop will be instilled.
  - Cataract surgery is usually considered fairly pain free. Paracetamol can be taken for mild pain or dull ache that is sometimes experienced.
  - Post-operative information leaflet must be given.

Phacoemulsification requires less stringent post-operative restrictions, swimming and driving being the two main activities to be avoided until advised otherwise, usually at the first post-operative outpatient visit. This is because swimming could cause irritation and eye rubbing response; and vision may be insufficient to meet the DVLA guidelines.

The patient may be seen and discharged by a health professional other than a doctor. This is usually a specially trained nurse or optometrist.

Patients will normally be advised to visit their optician two to four weeks after surgery for refraction and should they require glasses, the prescription will be given.

Listing for the second eye (if there is cataract) should be done as appropriate, often the assessment being undertaken over the telephone.

Cataract operations

The approach is via a limbal incision under a conjunctival flap or via a peripheral corneal incision.

Phacoemulsification

This is the most frequently used method with cataract in the adult patient. With phacoemulsification the lens is broken down by ultrasonic vibrations. This technique is becoming increasingly popular as it reduces the risk of expulsive haemorrhage and post-operative astigmatism (McNicholl, 1995) as the incision is smaller (as small as 3 mm in some cases) than that used in the operations described above. Suturing the wound is not required if it is properly sealed. A foldable intra-ocular lens is positioned in the posterior chamber. Alternatively, the wound is enlarged to accommodate a non-foldable lens implant.

Cool laser

This procedure is similar to phacoemulsification but uses 'cool laser' shock waves to fragment the lens. The fragments are aspirated. There are fewer intraoperative complications. As with the phacoemulsification technique, a lens implant is inserted (O'hEineachain, 2002).

Needling or lens aspiration

Needling or lens aspiration is performed on an infant or child under the age of 15 years. The cortex and nucleus of the lens are irrigated out through an incision in the anterior lens capsule, leaving the posterior capsule behind in order to prevent vitreous prolapse. At this age, the lens matter is soft enough to be aspirated.

The posterior lens capsule left behind often scleroses causing visual impairment when a capsulotomy will be performed using the Yag laser.

'Lensectomy' (phacofragmentation)

Lensectomy involves removing the entire lens and capsule and an anterior segment of the vitreous using specialised equipment. It is used for congenital cataracts and has the advantage of not requiring future capsulotomies.

Intracapsular lens extraction

In an intracapsular lens extraction, the entire lens plus its capsule is removed. An enzyme chymotripsin is introduced into the eye to dissolve the zonular fibres. The lens is then free of its attachments and can be removed from the eye by forceps or the cryoprobe. An anterior chamber intra-ocular lens will be implanted (see below). This procedure is rarely employed nowadays, but the nurse may encounter patients having had this type of surgery in the past.

Extracapsular lens extraction (ECCE)

In an extracapsular lens extraction the anterior lens capsule, the cortex and nucleus are removed, leaving the posterior lens capsule in place. The type of

incision made in the anterior lens capsule may vary, e.g. endocapsular, capsulorhexis. Following this type of surgery, cortical matter may proliferate on the intact posterior capsule, a condition requiring capsulotomy (see above). A posterior chamber intra-ocular lens will be implanted.

Aphakia

Correction of aphakia

Aphakia is the absence of the lens. Without the lens the eye becomes very hypermetropic, requiring some kind of lens replacement to enable the patient to see adequately. The only people who do not require correction of the aphakia are those who are very myopic in whom the absence of the lens causes the light rays to focus on the retina.

Aphakia causes loss of accommodation so patients will need correction for both near and distance vision. Following surgery, a degree of astigmatism will result, requiring correction as well.

Types of correction

Aphakia can be corrected using glasses, contact lenses or intra-ocular lenses.

Aphakic glasses

These glasses are rarely used nowadays. If they are worn, the patient needs to be made aware of the 'Jack-in-the box' effect they have on vision, objects appear to be jumping into the field of vision. They may be used in babies when contact lenses are unsuitable.

Contact lenses

Contact lenses are increasingly being superseded by intra-ocular lenses (see below) but nurses may meet patients who have had earlier surgery and wear contact lenses to correct their aphakia.

Use (in aphakia)

Unilateral or bilateral aphakia.

Advantages

Contact lenses:

- can be used for unilateral aphakia
- give a full field of vision
- can be used in babies and children
- only cause 7% magnification.

Disadvantages (see also Appendix 2)

- Patients have to become accustomed to wearing contact lenses; some may find them intolerable.
- Corneal abrasions and infections can result from contact lens wearing and from unclean lenses.
- Patients with arthritis cannot manipulate them but extended-wear lenses overcome this problem.
- The lenses are easily lost.
- They need scrupulous cleaning, especially soft contact lenses.
- People with bilateral aphakia may find difficulty in putting the first lens in because of poor sight in the other eye. Again, extended-wear lenses can overcome this.
- They are expensive for those who are not eligible to have them supplied by the NHS.
- They may not be suitable to be worn in some occupations, e.g. when working in a dusty environment.

Intra-ocular lenses

See Fig. 11.3.

Uses

Unilateral and bilateral aphakia.

Types

There are many different types of lenses made by the various companies. The following are examples what is available on the market.

Lenses are either rigid or foldable and come in a variety of materials including polymethylmethacrylate (PMMA) and acrylic. Some foldable lenses can be injected into the lens capsule. Where needed, multifocal and varifocal lenses can be used.

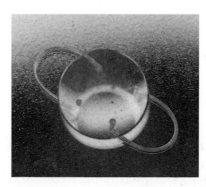

Fig. 11.3 An intra-ocular lens (IOL).

The lenses are designed specifically for either the anterior chamber or the posterior chamber.

Those for the anterior chamber, whilst they are rarely used now, are used following an intra-capsular extraction or if the posterior capsule ruptures during surgery.

Posterior chamber lenses are inserted into the posterior chamber of the eye following an extracapsular extraction, fitting into the posterior lens capsule which has been left behind. Newer lenses are being manufactured with 'laser ridges' to keep the lens away from the capsule to prevent the lens being damaged by the laser beam during a capsulotomy.

Folding lenses, e.g. Acrysoft, are used with phacoemulsification and are placed in the posterior capsule. They require a much smaller incision. Some are designed so that they can be injected into the capsule.

Selection

The choice of type and power of the IOL is determined by the surgeon who will take into account the needs of the patient. Such needs include the anatomy and physiology of the eye, whether the patient is myopic or hypermetropic. When the patient is having both eyes treated, there may be opportunity to alter focal length.

Advantages

- Full field of vision is attained 24 hours a day.
- They can be inserted at any time after the initial cataract extraction.
- No manual dexterity or manipulation is required by the wearer.
- They are suitable for workers in industry or those in a humid environment/occupation.
- Vision is good even without glasses. Bifocal intra-ocular lenses are available (Pearce, 1996), and are increasingly being used
- Posterior chamber intra-ocular lenses have been successfully implanted in children (Brady et al., 1995).
- Heparin-coated lenses can be used in patients with diabetes and also those who have repeated attacks of uveitis.

Disadvantages

- They can cause uveitis and glaucoma.
- They can dislocate.
- Anterior chamber lenses may cause bullous keratopathy.

Complications of cataract extraction

Modern cataract surgery gives good visual results and is a relatively safe procedure. However, complications do occur Kanski (2003):

Early

- zonular/posterior capsule rupture
- lens dislocation into vitreous
- vitreous loss
- wound gape/iris prolapse
- hyphaema
- vitreous/choroidal haemorrhage
- hypopyon
- endophthalmitis.

Late

- posterior capsular opacification, though occurs less frequently with the newer lenses
- uveitis
- cystoid macular oedema
- raised intra-ocular pressure
- dislocated/malpositioned intra-ocular lens (see Colour Plate 11)
- retinal detachment
- bullous keratopathy.

Dislocated lens

A total dislocation of the lens or a partial dislocation (subluxation) can occur.

This can be a result of trauma, it may be hereditary, or be associated with certain syndromes such as Marfan's syndrome. Vision will be blurred, but the degree of visual disturbance depends on the degree of dislocation. A partially dislocated lens can usually be seen through the pupil. A cataract may develop in the lens. A dislocated lens can cause uveitis or glaucoma by blocking either the posterior or anterior chambers.

If no complications occur, dislocated lenses are best left untreated. If complications do occur, treatment should be given to the complications before cataract extraction is attempted, as surgery in these instances is difficult.

Chapter 12
The Retina, Optic Nerve and Vitreous

The retina

The retina is composed of ten layers: one epithelial layer and nine neural layers. There is a potential space between the epithelial layer and neural layers which is significant in retinal detachment. The retina extends from the ora serrata anteriorly to the optic disc posteriorly where the nerve fibres leave the eye as the optic nerve.

Ten layers of the retina

These are illustrated in Fig. 12.1:

(1) The epithelial layer lies at the posterior of the structure beneath the choroid and contains varying amounts of melanin pigment. It absorbs light that is not picked up by the rods and cones.
(2) The receptor layer contains the rods and cones, which are the two main types of nerve endings in the retina. The rods, numbering about 120 million in each eye, are situated mainly at the periphery of the retina. They function in dim light. The cones, numbering around seven million in each eye, are situated at the centre of the retina and are concentrated, in particular, in the fovea of the macula. They function in bright light, pick up colours and make detailed vision possible.
(3) The external limiting membrane is like a sheet of wire netting and has a supportive function.
(4) The outer nuclear layer contains the nuclei of the rods and cones.
(5) The outer plexiform layer contains the axons of the rods and cones and the dendrites of the bipolar cells.
(6) The inner nuclear layer contains the nuclei of the bipolar cells.
(7) The inner plexiform layer contains the axons of bipolar cells and the dendrites of the ganglion cells.
(8) The ganglion cell layer contains the nuclei of the ganglion cells.
(9) The nerve fibre layer contains the axons of the ganglion cells which pass through the optic disc and lamina cibrosa to become continuous with the optic nerve.
(10) The internal limiting membrane has a supportive function.

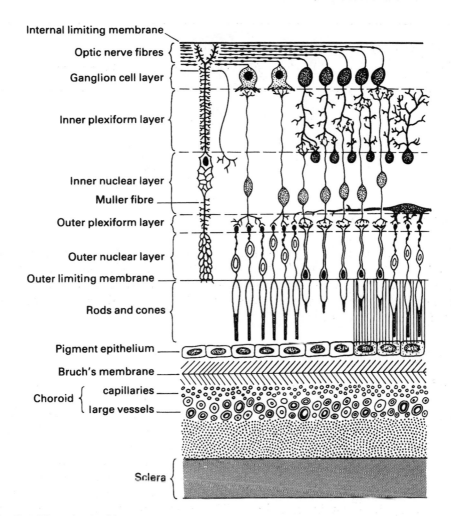

Fig. 12.1 Plan of retinal layers.

Layers 2 to 10 are known as the 'neural layers'.

Areas of the retina

Ora serrata: the anterior termination of the retina where the retinal pigment epithelial layer continues forwards to become the ciliary epithelium. The neural layer of the retina ends at the ora serrata.

Macula (Fig. 12.2): an area of the retina 1.5 mm in diameter situated 3 mm to the temporal side of the optic disc. It contains a high concentration of cones. In its centre is the fovea centralis, a slight depression where only cones are present. The other layers of the retina are absent here, causing a depression and making it thinner than the rest of the retina. The macula is the region of the retina where central precise vision takes place. It is not completely

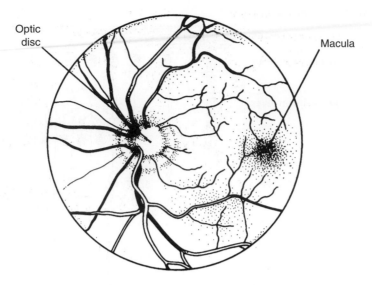

Fig. 12.2 Ophthalmoscopic view of the normal retina. (Reproduced with permission from Vaughan, D.G. & Asbury, T. (1983) *General Ophthalmology* (10th edn), Appleton & Lange.)

developed until six months after birth. No blood vessels cross the macula and it receives its blood supply entirely from the choriocapillaries.

Optic disc (Fig. 12.2): the area of the retina where the axons of the ganglion cells leave the eye through the lamina cribrosa to become continuous with the optic nerve. It therefore contains no nerve cells, so that vision cannot take place here. This is known as the 'blind spot'. The central retinal artery and vein pass through the optic disc. Its blood supply is from the posterior ciliary artery, a branch of the temporal artery.

Blood supply

The outer layers of the retina are supplied by the choriocapillaries of the choroid. The inner layers of the retina are supplied by the central retinal artery. The central retinal vein drains the venous blood.

Function of the retina

The retinal nerve cells pick up and transmit impulses from light rays reaching the retina. These impulses then travel via the optic pathways to the visual cortex where they are interpreted as sight (see Fig. 12.3). As light rays travel in straight lines they will fall on the diagonally opposite area of the retina from the object in view; for example, the light rays from an object viewed superiorly will fall on the inferior area of the retina. The same happens on the horizontal plane. The brain converts the image so it appears the right way up.

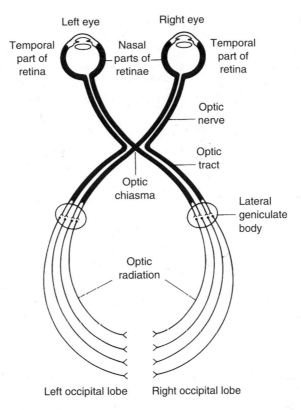

Fig. 12.3 Visual pathways. (Reprinted from Darling & Thorpe *Ophthalmic Nursing* (1981) Fig. 21, p. 74 by permission of the publisher Bailière Tindall Limited, London.)

The optic nerve

The optic nerve runs from the optic disc through the optic foramen to the optic chiasma where it becomes the optic tract. It is 5 cm in length and surrounded by pia mater, arachnoid mater and dura mater. Its blood supply is via the ophthalmic artery and vein.

The optic pathways

These are illustrated in Fig. 12.3. The optic nerve leaves each eye, passing through the optic foramen to the optic chiasma. From there the fibres from the left-hand side of each eye travel in the left-hand side of the brain and the right-hand fibres travel in the right-hand side of the brain. Thus the nasal fibres in the left eye cross at the chiasma to travel on the right side and the nasal fibres of the right eye cross to travel on the left side. The temporal fibres of each eye stay on their respective side. From the optic chiasma the fibres travel in the optic tracts to the lateral geniculate bodies where they pass into the optic radiations. From there the fibres pass to the visual area of the occipital cortex where sight is interpreted.

The vitreous

The vitreous fills the vitreous chamber which is the posterior segment of the eye lying between the lens and the retina (not to be confused with the posterior chamber).

It is a semi-gelatinous, transparent substance having no blood or nerve supply.

Composition

The vitreous is 98%–99% water; and 1%–2% hyaluronic acid and collagen fibres.

Attachments

The vitreous is attached more firmly to the underlying retina at the ora serrata and around the optic disc. Elsewhere it lies loosely against the retina. Sometimes it attaches itself to blood vessels, which could bleed if the vitreous pulled on them.

Functions of the vitreous

Refractions of light: the light rays travel in a converged manner through the vitreous towards the retina.

It maintains the shape of the eye; if it were lost, the eye would collapse. Vitreous cannot be replaced naturally by the eye.

Colour vision

The cones in the retina can be divided into three types: red, blue and green. Each of these types is sensitive to different light rays. The red absorb long waves, the green mid-length waves and the blue short waves. These differing wave lengths – or a combination of them – are interpreted as colour.

Rhodopsin

Rhodopsin is a photosensitive chemical present in the rods in the retina. In low-intensity light rhodopsin breaks down, taking a few moments to work and enabling the eye to adapt to dim light. When changing from low intensity light to bright light, it takes a few seconds to bleach the rhodopsin and enable the eye to adapt to bright light. Vitamin A is necessary for rhodopsin to function, thus a deficiency of vitamin A can lead to night blindness.

Conditions of the retina

Retinal detachment

Retinal detachment is a misnomer because it is not a detachment of the retina from the underlying choroid. It is, in fact, a separation of the epithelial layer from the neural layers of the retina. Because of the potential space between the first layer and the rest of the retina, it can become separated as a result of disease or trauma.

Causes

The neural retina can be either pulled, pushed or floated off the underlying epithelial layer.

Pulled off: the neural retina is pulled off the epithelial layer by vitreous traction. Vitreous traction occurs when new blood vessels have grown into the vitreous. The fragile vessels bleed and fibrous tissue forms in the healing process. These fibrous bands contract, pulling the neural layer away. Conditions causing this type of detachment are diabetes mellitus, retinopathy of prematurity, retinal haemorrhage and vitreous haemorrhage (see Colour Plates 12 and 13).

Pushed off: a lesion behind the retina pushes the retina forwards, causing fluid or exudate to separate the layers of the retina. Conditions causing this type of detachment are choroidal tumours, choroidal haemorrhage, choroiditis and retinopathies.

Floated off: if a tear or hole appears in the retina, subretinal fluid or vitreous fluid enters the hole, floating the neural layers off the epithelial layer. Tears in the retina occur following trauma, in high myopes, retinal degeneration (see p. 176) and aphakia. The tears usually occur in the periphery or equator of the retina.

Patient's needs

- Relief of symptoms:
  - Flashing lights (photopsia) – caused by the separating layers of the retina stimulating the rods and cones.
  - Floaters – a sudden increase in the number of floaters in the vision, or a shower of floaters, occurs. These are small haemorrhages, usually from retinal vessels.
  - Field loss – as the retina separates, the affected part causes loss of vision in the corresponding visual field. It must be remembered that the visual field loss is opposite to the detachment; for example, if the upper half of the retina is detached, the visual loss would be the lower half of the visual field. It is important to prevent the macula from detaching, as the visual prognosis following this occurrence is not good. The separated macula will be denied its blood supply from the choriocapillaries and will therefore become anoxic. Unfortunately the

commonest site for a detachment is in the superior temporal area causing an inferior nasal visual field loss. This area of the visual field is occluded to some extent by the nose, the vision in the other eye compensating for it. Therefore field loss in this area is not noticed as quickly as field loss in another area. Also a superior detachment can progress more rapidly due to gravity and the danger of a macular detachment is therefore greater.

- Admission to hospital for bed rest and pre- and post-operative care.
- Surgery to re-attach the retina.

Nursing action

- Take an accurate history.
- Inform the doctor of the patient's history and type of visual loss.
- Instil prescribed mydriatic drops as prescribed or as per PGD, for oph-thalmoscopic examination of the fundus.
- Admit patient to the ward.
- Give pre-operative care:
  - ○ Bed rest, to prevent further detachment occurring.
  - ○ Dependent positioning: this is decided, to some extent, by the doctor's wishes and the site of the detachment. The rationale is to position the patient so that the detachment lies dependently against its underlying epithelial layer, encouraging the subretinal fluid to be absorbed and re-attachment to occur.
  - ○ Instil prescribed mydriatic drops regularly to maintain mydriasis so that a good fundal examination can be carried out. This is performed using an indirect ophthalmoscope and a 20 dioptre lens to obtain an accurate diagram of the retina, including tears, holes, detached and attached areas, and the presence of subretinal fluid. This helps the surgeon at the time of operation. The other eye is also dilated and inspected. Retinopathies, degenerations, and myopia can affect both eyes. Problems in the other eye must be noted and treated if present, often using laser or cryotherapy prophylactically.
- Give post-operative care:
  - (a) Eye care:
    - (i) The lids and conjunctiva are usually swollen following retinal detachment because of the amount of movement of the eye that is necessary during the operation.
    - (ii) The cornea must be noted for its clarity; if it is cloudy, this could indicate ischaemia of the anterior segment of the eye caused by the encirclement band being too tight (see below).
    - (iii) The pupil will remain dilated.
    - (iv) Antibiotic, mydriatic and steroid drops, non-steroidal anti-inflammatory drops may be prescribed.
  - (b) General care: the patient may be nursed in a dependent position fol-lowing surgery. This is especially important following vitrectomy, when the injected gas or air bubble must be uppermost to put

pressure on the detached retina (see below). Analgesia will need to be given regularly as ocular pain will be experienced by most patients. It must be ascertained that the cause of pain is not raised pressure due to anterior segment ischaemia (see above).

Types of retinal detachment surgery

The eye is not opened for detachment surgery, the approach being from the outside over the sclera, apart from a vitrectomy in which case the eye is opened.

Cryotherapy, laser or photocoagulation is performed to seal holes or tears by setting up a local inflammatory reaction and thereby preventing fluid seeping between the retinal layers. Holes and tears, if present, must be sealed during detachment operations for this surgery to be successful (see Colour Plate 14).

Plombage or scleral buckling: a silastic sponge or 'plomb' (a small square of inert material) is sutured onto the sclera over the site of the hole, causing an indentation and bringing the separated layers of the retina together.

Encirclement: a silicone band is positioned around the globe, underneath the extra-ocular muscles. This enables greater indentation to occur and is used where there is a large area of detachment or multiple holes.

Drainage of subretinal fluid must be performed at the time of each of the above surgical procedures to allow the separated layers to realign.

Vitrectomy may be performed in certain circumstances (see below).

Complications

- Early:
  o Subretinal fluid may continue to accumulate between the layers of the retina. This must be removed if spontaneous reabsorption does not occur in order to prevent further detachment occurring and to aid re-attachment.
  o Ischaemia of the anterior segment of the eye following encirclement if the band is too tight.
- Late:
  o Infection of the plomb or band, in which case removal is necessary.
  o Extrusion of the plomb: the plomb may become loose and work its way to the surface under the conjunctiva.

Vitrectomy

Vitrectomy is performed for the following conditions:

- giant tears
- retinal detachment with scar formation
- macula hole
- fibrovascular tissue in diabetic retinopathy (see Colour Plate 15)

- dislocated lens (subluxation – see Colour Plate 11)
- foreign body in posterior segment
- penetrating injury
- vitreous tap for microscopy.

Vitreous cannot be replaced naturally. One of the following substances is used as replacement material:

- Gas, e.g. SF_6 (Sulphur Hexafluoride), $C_3 F_8$ (Perfluoropropane): the patient cannot see through the gas until it has been absorbed and this takes two to three weeks.
- Silicone oil: the patient can see through the oil but it makes the eye hypermetropic. Silicone oil is not absorbed and is removed later.
- Air: this is absorbed within 24 to 36 hours.
- Gas and air mixture.
- $C_{10} F_{18}$ (perfluorodecaline): this is a heavy liquid which is not absorbed.

Aqueous will gradually fill the vitreous chamber to replace the above substances as they are absorbed (except the oil and $C_{10} F_{18}$).

In order to carry out a vitrectomy, the vitreous chamber/posterior segment is approached via three entry ports at the ora serrata (pars plana) to prevent damage to the retina. The vitreous is broken up and aspirated out of the eye. All instruments entering the vitreous chamber are 27 gauge in size. Up to 90% of the vitreous can be removed.

Complications of vitrectomy surgery

- Cataract formation.
- Oil in the anterior segment.
- Emulsified oil in the anterior chamber or between the main bubble and the retina.

The bubble will expand when flying. Patients are advised not to fly if the bubble is more than 10% of the volume of the eye.

Additional post-operative nursing care

- Eye care: observe the entry sites in the sclera for bleeding and gaping.
- Post-operative positioning: the head must be positioned so that the gas, air or oil is lying against the hole/detachment. If a macular hole has been repaired it is especially important that the patient is positioned face down for the majority of time for ten days to two weeks after surgery. During this time they are at risk of the complications or immobility, including pressure sores. The patient can have five or ten minutes 'relief' from positioning every hour, depending on the surgeon's wishes.

Central retinal artery occlusion

Central retinal artery occlusion is considered an ophthalmic emergency because instituting treatment within two hours of occurrence may restore the vision which would otherwise be permanently lost. This condition occurs suddenly, without warning, causing painless loss of vision. It is rare, usually only affecting one eye. It is caused by an embolus or thrombus due to arteriosclerosis, mitral stenosis, carotid insufficiency or temporal arteritis and as a complication of thyroid eye disease.

Signs

- The eye will look white.
- Visual acuity will be reduced to count fingers, hand movements or perception of light only.
- The fundus looks pale due to oedema obliterating the normal red reflex. The macula stands out as a 'cherry red spot', this area being unaffected by the oedema as the retina here is thinner (see p. 161) and no blood vessels cross it. The red reflex from the underlying choroid can therefore be seen. The retinal arteries are small, containing segmented columns of blood called 'cattle tracking'. The retinal veins appear normal.

Patient's needs

- Prompt medical attention for diagnosis to be made and treatment commenced.
- Investigation into the cause and relevant treatment given if necessary.

Nursing priorities

- Inform the medical staff immediately of the patient's visual acuity and sudden onset of symptoms.
- Prepare equipment for treatment (see below).

Nursing action

- Instil prescribed mydriatic for ophthalmoscopic examination of the retina, so that the diagnosis can be established.
- Prepare the patient and the equipment that the doctor may require to try to restore vision. The following methods can be employed, the aim of the treatment being to dislodge the embolus or thrombus or increase the oxygen supply to the retina:
  o An anterior chamber paracentesis – a needle is introduced into the anterior chamber to reduce the intra-ocular pressure suddenly.
  o Give 500 mg acetazolamide intravenously to reduce the intra-ocular pressure.
  o massage over the globe.

○   give 100% oxygen.

○   ask the patient to blow into a paper bag to raise the carbon dioxide levels in the blood, which, in turn, will stimulate more oxygen to be produced.

○   give a vasodilator, e.g. talazoline hydrochloride (Priscol).

The nurse should not institute any of these measures without instructions from the doctor, as the diagnosis of sudden visual loss must be differentiated from that of a retinal detachment (see p. 165), temporal arteritis (see p. 225) or central retinal vein occlusion (see below).

* Check blood pressure and test a specimen of urine.

If sight is not restored by any of these methods, there is no other treatment available. If sight is already poor in the other eye, the patient will need help and advice from the social services department (see p. 3).

Central retinal vein occlusion

Central retinal vein occlusion is a more common occurrence than retinal artery occlusion. It also affects one eye, the visual loss being sudden but usually less devastating. It is caused by hypertension, diabetes mellitus, arteriosclerosis, glaucoma and thyroid eye disease.

Signs

* The eye will be white.
* The visual acuity will have dropped to 6/36 or less.
* The fundus will be red and swollen, with dilated and tortuous veins. Retinal haemorrhages will be present.

Patient's needs

* Prompt medical attention so that a diagnosis can be made and treatment commenced.
* Investigation into the cause, and appropriate treatment given if necessary.

Nursing priority

Inform medical staff immediately of the patient's visual acuity and history of sudden onset.

Nursing action

* Instil the prescribed mydriatic drop so that the fundus can be examined and a diagnosis made.
* Measure blood pressure and test a specimen of urine.

- Ensure the patient understands the instructions for the investigations.
- Ensure he understands the treatment, which may be one of the following:
  - ○ oral steroids
  - ○ dipyridamole and aspirin to prevent the 'stickiness' of the platelets
  - ○ photocoagulation or laser treatment to coagulate bleeding retinal vessels.

Prognosis

Vision may recover spontaneously over several weeks or it may remain unchanged.

Complications

- Vitreous haemorrhage (see p. 184) from new blood vessels growing in the ischaemic retina which bleed. This could cause a retinal detachment.
- Thrombotic glaucoma (see p. 144). Neovascularisation from the ischaemic retina occurs in the iris and anterior chamber angle, blocking the drainage angle.
- Atrophy of the retina and optic nerve from ischaemia of these structures (see p. 183).
- Cystoid macular oedema (see p. 181).

Retinal haemorrhage

Retinal haemorrhage can occur in any layer of the retina, appearing as flame-shaped areas or as round blots. It can collect in the pre-retinal space between the retina and the vitreous.

Causes

- Vascular conditions, e.g. arteriosclerosis and hypertension (see below).
- Blood diseases such as anaemia, leukaemia and sickle-cell anaemia.
- Trauma.
- Retinopathies due to diabetes, hypertension, nephritis and toxaemia of pregnancy (see below).

The treatment is that of the cause and bed rest to settle the haemorrhage. Vitrectomy may be required (see p. 167).

Retinopathies

Retinopathies are caused by diabetes mellitus, hypertension, renal disease and toxaemia of pregnancy. The result is a combination of retinal degeneration and inflammation.

1: Diabetic retinopathy

Diabetic retinopathy is the leading cause of blindness in the western world in the under 65 year-olds. The National Service Framework for Diabetes (2002) states that diabetes is the leading cause of blindness in people of working age. Diabetes, being essentially a vascular disease, affects the blood vessels of the retina. Until recently it was thought that diabetic retinopathy occurred after 20 years or so regardless of the diabetic control. Recent research (The Diabetes Control and Complications Trial Research Group, 1995) indicates strongly that good control does prevent ocular and other diabetic complications. Puberty adversely affects the onset and subsequent development of retinopathy (Jose et al., 1994).

The complications of diabetes such as renal impairment, vascular complications such as strokes and coronary heart disease, amputation can have a devastating effect on the patients and their families. Effects such as the physical, psychological and material well-being have all been cited in the National Service Framework for Diabetes (2002). Diabetes also has a major impact on the health and social services. Five percent of the total NHS resources have been used for the care of diabetic patients (National Service Framework for Diabetes, 2002).

To halt the progression of diabetic retinopathy, it is extremely important that any sight-threatening diabetic retinopathy is detected early and all patients with diabetes be screened, and where appropriate laser treatment instituted. Patients suffering from visual impairment should be supported through the use of low visual aids, psychological support, financial support, and from voluntary organisations such as Royal National Institute of the Blind and diabetic retinopathy self help groups.

There are five stages of diabetic retinopathy:

- background retinopathy (see Colour Plate 13);
- maculopathy;
- pre-proliferative retinopathy;
- proliferative retinopathy (see Colour Plate 12);
- advanced retinopathy.

Background retinopathy

Background retinopathy occurs in most diabetics about 20 years after the onset of the disease and therefore can affect all age groups from late teens onwards. It usually gives no symptoms to the patient until the macula is involved with resulting impairment of central vision. The patient may complain of glare due to the light rays being scattered by the oedematous retina.

Signs

The fundus has a typical picture of dots, blots and hard waxy exudates. The dots are micro-aneurysms. The blots are small haemorrhages. The hard waxy exudates are leakages of lipids from the haemorrhaging blood vessels. A ring of exudates around the macula suggests maculopathy (see below).

Patient's needs

- Annual medical ophthalmic check-ups to assess the degree of retinopathy.
- Control of cholesterol levels by giving Clofibrate tablets 500 mg three times a day.
- The patient may require advice on his treatment and diet from a diabetic clinic.

Nursing action

Care for the patient in the outpatient department when attending for check-ups.

Maculopathy

Maculopathy is the main cause of visual impairment in non-insulin dependent diabetics. There are four types:

- Focal/exudative: this can be treated by laser.
- Cystoid/diffuse: this is difficult to treat by laser.
- Ischaemic: cannot be treated.
- Mixed: can be treated by laser.

Patient's needs

- Diagnosis of which type of maculopathy is present.
- Treatment with the argon laser as appropriate.
- Relief from central visual impairment.

Nursing action

- Prepare the patient for fundal fluorescein angiography (see p. 46).
- Prepare the patient for laser treatment (see p. 48). Laser treatment seals the leaking blood vessels around the macula, thereby reducing the production of hard exudates. The laser beam is directed at the macula but must avoid the fovea itself, as loss of central vision would result if this was hit by the beam.

Pre-proliferative retinopathy

Pre-proliferative retinopathy may develop in eyes with background retinopathy only.

Signs

The retina is ischaemic which causes:

- cotton wool spots – ischaemic nerve fibre layer;
- dilation, beading, looping of blood vessels;
- arteriole narrowing;
- large dark blot haemorrhages.

There is no specific treatment unless the eye is the only seeing eye, in which case laser treatment is applied.

There are no symptoms but the patient's eyes need careful observation as they are prone to develop proliferative retinopathy.

Proliferative retinopathy

This is the main cause of visual impairment in insulin dependent diabetics. It occurs sooner, after diagnosis of the disease, in non-insulin dependent diabetics, possibly because the disease has gone on for longer undetected. The body's natural response to the ischaemic retina is to liberate a vasoprolific factor which stimulates the formation of new blood vessels to try to overcome the lack of oxygen to the structures involved.

The problem with newly formed blood vessels is that they are very fragile and bleed easily. In proliferative retinopathy these blood vessels grow into the vitreous and they bleed, causing vitreous haemorrhage. Eventually traction bands of fibrous tissue form which pull on the retina causing a retinal detachment. These new vessels can be seen easily on ophthalmoscopy and angiography.

The aim of the treatment is to prevent the neovascularisation occurring. The laser beam is applied to the retina. Dead retina will not encourage new vessel growth. Thus the retina is peppered with small areas of scotomas from laser treatment. These scotomas appear to cause little visual impairment to the patient. Vitrectomy will remove the haemorrhage as well as the scaffold that the new vessels grow into.

Patient's needs

- Treatment of proliferative retinopathy by the laser to prevent further deterioration.
- Treatment of the vitreous haemorrhage.
- Guidance around the hospital if visual acuity is poor.

Nursing action

- Prepare the patient for laser treatment (see p. 48).
- Admit the patient to hospital and prepare for vitrectomy (see p. 167).
- Assist the severely visually handicapped patient.

Advanced retinopathy

This is the end result of uncontrolled proliferative retinopathy and results in blindness.

Signs

- Persistent vitreous haemorrhage.
- Retinal detachment.
- 'Burnt-out stage' when no new vessels are stimulated to grow because the retina has become anoxic due to there being more fibrous than vascular tissue.
- Neovascular or thrombotic glaucoma due to new vessels growing in the anterior chamber angle obstructing the outflow of aqueous.

Patient's needs

- Vitrectomy if not performed previously.
- Treatment of neovascular glaucoma.
- Management of visual impairment.

Nursing action

- Prepare the patient for vitrectomy (see p. 167).
- Assist in the treatment of glaucoma.
- Instruct the patient to instil beta-blockers, e.g. Betoptic, twice a day and take acetazolamide 250 mg four times a day.
- Prepare the patient for laser treatment to new vessels in angle and/or for trabeculoplasty (see 'Laser treatment' on p. 142).
- Prepare the patient for trabeculectomy (see 'Surgical treatment' on p. 142) or insertion of a filtering tube, e.g. Molteno, if above measures have failed.
- Inform the patient about services available and refer to social worker and low visual aid clinic as appropriate.

2: Hypertensive retinopathy (including renal disease and toxaemia of pregnancy)

Hypertensive retinopathy is caused by primary hypertension and hypertension secondary to renal disease and toxaemia of pregnancy. Patients usually have no symptoms until the haemorrhages and exudates affect the macula with resulting central field involvement.

There are four stages, graded according to their severity:

- Grade I: there is generalised arterial constriction which gives the fundal picture of 'silver' or 'copper wiring' due to increased light reflex from the thickened arterial walls.

- Grade II. There is arteriovenous 'nipping' due to arteriosclerosis. The thickened arterial wall obscures the vein lying beneath it.
- Grade III. In grade III haemorrhages and exudates appear. Flame-shaped haemorrhages follow the nerve fibres and are superficial. Round haemorrhages lie deeper in the retinal layers. Exudates are not in fact exudates as such but are white 'fluffy' areas of infarcted nerve fibres due to ischaemia.
- Grade IV. All the above signs are present plus papilloedema. Renal failure will probably have occurred and vision is grossly impaired. Characteristically in renal retinopathy there is a well-defined star appearance of exudates at the macula.

Patient's needs

- Regular ophthalmic check-ups including fundal fluorescein angiography to document any changes in the retinal blood vessels.
- Treatment of the underlying cause. Referral to a physician may be necessary. If the toxaemia of pregnancy is severe, the pregnancy may need to be terminated to save the mother's sight and life.

Nursing action

- Assist the patient in the outpatient department.
- Measure blood pressure and test urine specimen.
- Prepare the patient for a fundal fluorescein angiography (see p. 46).

Prognosis

If the underlying cause is kept under control, visual prognosis is fairly good. Once the macular area becomes involved vision deteriorates. A severe retinopathy results in poor visual acuity and an accompanying poor prognosis. A complication of toxaemic retinopathy is a retinal detachment (see p. 165).

Retinal degenerations

Degenerations of the retina occur around its periphery. Some are significant in that they may cause retinal detachment (see p. 165). These are lattice and snail-track degeneration and acquired retinoschisis. Other degenerations – such as snowflake, paving stone and honeycomb – are insignificant, causing no ophthalmic complication.

Retinitis pigmentosa

Retinitis pigmentosa is a hereditary degeneration of the retinal nerve cells affecting one in 2500. The heredity is variable, resulting in varying degrees of severity. The autosomal and X-linked recessive forms are severe with symptoms starting in teenage years. The autosomal dominant form is less severe with symptoms occurring in later adult life. The rods are slowly destroyed, initially affecting the peripheral retina causing night blindness. Eventually the whole retina is affected when tunnel vision results.

An electroretinogram is performed to diagnose the condition. Later colour vision is affected. Eventually even the macula may be involved, causing total blindness. Cataracts may develop.

On ophthalmoscopy, the retina is peppered with black pigment. There is no known treatment. Management is aimed at improving visual impairment with low visual aids, pinhole spectacles and eye shields.

Couples should receive genetic counselling before starting a family if one of them is affected.

Retinopathy of prematurity

The retinal blood vessels' development is not complete until the month after birth. Therefore a baby born prematurely will have an incompletely developed retinal blood supply. If the baby is given a high concentration of oxygen in an incubator, the stimulus for the continuing development of the retinal vessels is withdrawn. When the baby is removed from the oxygen supply, the retina is receiving insufficient oxygen and it becomes anoxic, resulting in proliferation of new vessels.

Although the oxygen now delivered to incubators is monitored closely, and must continue to be so, the condition is still occurring. It is thought to be due more to the prematurity or low birth weight of the baby than to the concentration of oxygen (Duker & Tolentino, 1991). O'Conner & Glasper (1995) suggest it is a multifactoral condition.

There are five stages of the disease. Stages 1 and 2 generally regress without treatment. The other stages are treated by laser to decrease the proliferation. Visual prognosis tends to be poor. Screening of premature and low birth weight babies is essential at approximately six to nine weeks after birth.

Retinal tumour: retinoblastoma

A retinoblastoma is a retinal tumour occurring in children under the age of five years. It is very rare but highly malignant, occurring in one in 20 000 live births. It usually only affects one eye, but in 30% of cases is bilateral, both growths being primary tumours. There may be a family history of retinoblastoma.

Signs

- A white pupil is noted, the tumour showing through the pupil instead of the normal red choroidal reflex. A white pupil may also be a sign of a cataract.
- The child may have a squint because he will not be using the affected eye for seeing and it will deviate inwards.

Treatment

The eye will be enucleated (see Chapter 15), unless the tumour is small, in which case photocoagulation, cryotherapy, laser or radiotherapy treatment will be used, preserving the eye and maybe some sight. External beam radiation providing a lens sparing technique results in less damage to the eye than whole eye radiation (Toma et al., 1995). If the child presents with bilateral tumours, the sight of one eye will be preserved as far as possible without endangering the child's life. The eye with the smallest tumour will be treated by one of the methods mentioned.

Careful watch must be kept on an unaffected fellow eye. If a tumour occurs in it, it must be treated promptly as above to destroy the tumour and preserve as much sight as possible.

Siblings must be checked for the presence of a retinoblastoma and children of surviving sufferers must be examined at birth and observed until the age of five years.

Prognosis

The earlier the diagnosis is made and treatment instituted, the higher the chance of preventing metastases. An untreated tumour spreads within the eye, causing it to become glaucomatous. From the eye malignant cells track back into the orbit and brain via the optic nerve and can metastasise into the liver and elsewhere in the body. A late diagnosis will result in a poorer prognosis for the child's life.

Cytomegalovirus retinitis

Cytomegalovirus (CMV) is a common member of the herpes virus family, usually remaining dormant unless the person is immuno-compromised. Cytomegalovirus retinitis is the commonest opportunistic infection in people with AIDS, affecting 20–30% of sufferers (Engstrom & Holland, 1995). As it is a progressive disease, it can result in severe visual impairment. Recurrence of the disease heralds a particularly poor visual prognosis.

Signs

Retinal haemorrhages and exudates are present which progress to become necrotic eventually involving the optic disc. Retinal detachment can occur as can cataracts.

Patient's needs

- Diagnosis of the disease.
- Medical or surgical treatment as appropriate.
- Professional counselling/referral if diagnosis of AIDS is made in the ophthalmic department.

Nursing action

- Assist in diagnostic tests: ophthalmoscopy, fundal photography.
- Explain the different treatment modalities:
  - ○ Ganciclovir (dihydroxypropoxymethyl guanine – DHPG)
    Induction: 5 mg/kg body weight intravenously twice a day for two to three weeks. Maintenance: single daily dose of 5 mg/kg body weight intravenously every day; or 6 mg/kg body weight intravenously for five days a week; or 3 g per day oral Ganciclovir.
  - ○ Foscarnet (trisodium phosphonoformate)
    Induction: 60 mg/kg body weight three times a day for two to three weeks. Maintenance: 90–120 mg/kg body weight intravenously daily indefinitely.
    Maintenance treatment has to be given indefinitely as the virus lies dormant. Despite maintenance, recurrences are common. Ganciclovir and Foscarnet treat the CMV retinitis but have no effect on the AIDS itself. Drugs that treat the AIDS, e.g. AZT, cannot be given concurrently with Ganciclovir as the combined drugs are too toxic to bone marrow. Drugs similar to AZT are on trial that cause less bone marrow toxicity. Ganciclovir implants in the vitreous are being tried (Martin et al., 1994).
- Prepare the patient for retinal detachment surgery/vitrectomy (see p. 167).
- Refer the patient to counselling/AIDS service as appropriate.
- Employ infection control procedures according to local policies. It must be remembered that the HIV virus is very weak and does not survive outside the body. Although it has been isolated in tears, large quantities are required for transmission of the virus.

Prognosis

Patients being treated for CMV retinitis in one eye rarely get it in the fellow eye (Jabs et al., 1989), whereas untreated patients have an incidence of 60% occurrence in the fellow eye. Thus if one eye is blind from CMV retinitis, treatment will continue to protect the other eye.

Conditions of the macula

Age-related macular degeneration

Age-related macular degeneration is a bilateral condition affecting the cones in the macular region, in old age (see Colour Plate 16). There are two types of age-related macular degeneration – dry and wet. It is thought that there might be a hereditary element and that myopia may be a predisposing factor. There is gradual loss of central vision, but peripheral vision is retained so that the patient will always be able to retain his 'navigational' vision. The loss of central vision causes much distress to the patients. They are unable to recognise people because they cannot see their faces clearly, they cannot see the bus numbers, sign for their pensions, watch television clearly or read. They need continual reassurance that they will not go completely blind.

Dry (atrophic or non-neovascular) macular degeneration

The dry form of macular degeneration is more common than the wet macular degeneration accounting for 85% to 90% of all age macular degeneration. It is associated with small, round, white-yellow lesions in the macula called drusen. There is currently no treatment for dry macular degeneration.

Wet (choroidal neovascularisation) macular degeneration

Wet, age-related macular degeneration accounts for 10% to 15% of all age-related macular degeneration and is characterised by the development of abnormal blood vessels beneath the retinal pigment epithelium layer of the retina. Significant central visual loss is also much greater than the dry form of macular degeneration. Many studies have been done to identify the risk factors for age related macular degeneration such as age (usually over the age of 50), race (more prevalent in white women), smoking, hypertension, genetics and menopause. The role of vitamins and antioxidants in the prevention of macular degeneration is a much-debated issue.

Patient's needs

- Investigations into type of degeneration.
- Photodynamic therapy (laser treatment) if applicable.
- Psychological and social effects.
- Where appropriate, low visual aids to improve vision and quality of life.

Nursing action

- Prepare the patient for fundal fluorescein angiography (see p. 46) and indocyanine green (ICG) if requested (see p. 47).
- Prepare the patient for photodynamic therapy (see p. 49)

Low visual aid

Assist the patient with explanations and demonstrations in the aids available. These include low visual aids which are obtained from the optician and which may be one or more of the following, depending on the individual's needs:

- Magnifying glasses – these can be hand-held in varying shapes and sizes or made with stands to sit on the page and be moved along the line of print.
- Telescopic lenses – these lenses are attached to spectacles and the item to be read must be held close to the eye. This takes time to become accustomed to and can prove quite awkward for the patient. Some telescopes are illuminated with a battery.
- A good light from an anglepoise-type lamp positioned correctly over the shoulder can make a lot of difference to central vision.
- Special aids are available to assist in signing pension books, etc. These are cardboard cut-outs which can be placed over the area to be written on, guiding the patient to sign in the correct place.
- Magnification using computer screens may be useful.

Remember to keep reassuring the patient that peripheral navigation vision will not be lost. He may wish to be registered as blind or partially sighted (see p. 2).

Central serous retinopathy

Central serous retinopathy is a maculopathy affecting a younger age group than age-related macular degeneration. The cause is unknown and occurs in the 25–40 years age group, affecting men more than women. The sufferers tend to have an anxious disposition. The patients complain of a sudden painless loss of central vision, for example down to 6/18 with a central blur. The macula is elevated with a diagnostic light reflex around the macula.

The patient will be asked to read the Amsler grid to assess the size and position of the central blur. A fundal fluorescein angiogram (see p. 46) will highlight the leaking of serous fluid from the choriocapillaries through the defect in the pigment epithelium. Laser treatment can be applied to seal the leaking vessels. The condition usually resolves itself within two to four months.

Cystoid macular oedema/degeneration

Cystoid macular oedema/degeneration is a rare condition causing loss of central vision. The oedema results from leakages of fluid from the retinal capillaries which infiltrate the retinal layers around the macula. It occurs gradually and can be caused by diabetic retinopathy, retinal vein occlusion, uveitis and following intra-ocular surgery when the exact causative mechanism is unknown.

A fundal fluorescein angiogram shows the leaking vessels forming a petal appearance around the macula. The condition usually regresses spontaneously but there may be permanent visual loss, especially following cataract extraction. Patients who experience slow visual deterioration following intra-ocular surgery may have this condition.

Conditions of the optic nerve

Optic neuritis

Optic neuritis is an inflammation, degeneration or demyelinisation of the optic nerve at the optic disc, causing sudden loss of vision.

Causes

- Demyelinising diseases such as multiple sclerosis.
- Systemic infections. Viral infections such as poliomyelitis, influenza, mumps and measles.
- Lebers disease is a hereditary inflammation of the optic nerve affecting men aged between 20 and 30 years. Vision is not totally lost but there is no known treatment.
- Local extension of inflammatory disease such as sinusitis, meningitis, orbital cellulitis.
- Toxic amblyopia is caused by a high intake of tobacco, alcohol, quinine and chloroquine.
- No cause may be discovered.

Signs

- The optic disc is pale and oedematous with blurred disc margins.
- The large retinal veins are distended.

Patient's needs

- Diagnosis of the cause of the optic neuritis.
- Institution of treatment.

Nursing priority

- Inform the medical staff of the patient's sudden loss of vision.

Nursing action

- Record blood pressure and test a specimen of urine.
- Instil prescribed mydriatic, as per prescription or PGD for ophthalmoscopic examination.
- Ensure the patient understands the blood tests and X-rays necessary to determine the cause.

Treatment

- The underlying cause must be treated if possible. Toxic amblyopia is treated by total abstinence of the offending toxin. Patients receiving

chloroquine as treatment for rheumatoid arthritis or systemic lupus erythematosus must have regular ophthalmic examinations.
- Systemic steroids.

Prognosis

The visual loss is usually maximal within several days of onset. It will then begin to improve two to three weeks afterwards and a gradual recovery occurs over several months. Recurrent attacks can cause permanent damage eventually.

Retrobulbar neuritis

Retrobulbar neuritis is inflammation of the optic nerve occurring behind the optic disc. This means that changes in the nerve cannot be seen with the ophthalmoscope. The patient's vision suddenly diminishes. It has been said that retrobulbar neuritis is a condition where the patient sees nothing out of the eye and the doctor sees nothing (abnormal) in the eye.

The causes are similar to those of optic neuritis. The treatment is that of the cause plus systemic and maybe retrobulbar steroids.

Optic nerve atrophy

Atrophy of the optic nerve can result from any of a number of causes:

- vascular – central retinal artery and vein occlusion
- degeneration and resulting atrophy from retinal diseases, such as retinitis pigmentosa, and systemic diseases, such as multiple sclerosis
- papilloedema
- optic and retrobulbar neuritis
- pressure on the optic nerve from aneurysms, glaucoma, tumours and orbital disease
- toxic conditions, such as toxic amblyopia
- metabolic disease, such as diabetes mellitus
- trauma.

The signs of optic atrophy are a pale optic disc and loss of pupillary reaction to light.

The visual loss is gradual resulting in varying degrees from complete blindness to scotoma, depending on the cause. The cause must be elicited so that it can be treated.

The prognosis is usually poor. Optic atrophy caused by pressure may improve once the pressure has been relieved.

Conditions of the vitreous

Vitreous floaters

Vitreous floaters are small opacities in the vitreous that can stimulate the retina by casting a shadow on it. The mind projects the corresponding dark form onto the appropriate field of vision. Most people experience a mild degree of vitreous floaters. When looking at a uniform background they will see minute specks in their field of vision. As long as these specks move with eye movement they are not potentially dangerous.

However, an increase in the number of floaters occurs as one grows older and the vitreous gel degenerates, a condition known as syneresis. Myopes are also prone to an increase in the number of their floaters. There is no treatment and people often learn to live with the floaters which they may refer to as their 'friends'.

Vitreous floaters become significant in the following circumstances.

- A sudden onset of 'cobweb' or 'spider' in the vision indicates that the vitreous attachment at the optic disc has become detached, resulting in a vitreous detachment (see below).
- Flashes of light indicate that the liquefied vitreous, swirling around on eye movement, is putting traction on the retina. This could progress to a retinal detachment.
- A sudden crop of black floaters indicates the presence of a retinal tear with an associated vitreous haemorrhage. This may progress to a vitreous detachment followed by a retinal detachment.

Thus it can be seen that vitreous floaters may indicate further vitreous and retinal conditions.

Posterior vitreous detachment

Posterior vitreous detachment occurs with the degeneration of the vitreous. The vitreous detaches from its attachment around the optic disc. A 'spider's web' or 'cobweb' is noticed in the vision and a sudden increase in vitreous floaters occurs. Flashing lights may also be seen as the detaching vitreous stimulates the rods and cones.

Vitreous detachment may cause vitreous haemorrhage, retinal tears and retinal detachment and should be investigated.

Patients are often very concerned about these symptoms. Information about this condition should be given to them.

Vitreous haemorrhage

Vitreous haemorrhage may vary in degree from minimal bleeding, in which case the patient notices a few more floaters, to a massive bleed obscuring sight suddenly so the patient can only see light.

Causes

- Trauma.
- Vascular disorders such as hypertension, leukaemia, neovascularisation especially in diabetic retinopathy, and following a central retinal vein occlusion.
- Vitreous detachment.

Signs

- The fundal picture will vary according to the size of the haemorrhage, from small opacities floating in the vitreous to a total haemorrhage obscuring the fundus.

Patient's needs

- Diagnosis of cause of haemorrhage in order that treatment can be instituted.
- Bed rest to assist absorption of haemorrhage.
- Preparation for vitrectomy.

Nursing action

- If visual loss has occurred suddenly, the medical staff should be informed immediately.
- Instil prescribed mydriatic drops for ophthalmoscopy.
- Admit the patient to the ward if the haemorrhage is severe enough to warrant bed rest in hospital.
- Give pre-operative care if vitrectomy is to be performed.
- If the patient is not to be admitted, ensure that he understands the importance of resting at home.
- Give post-vitrectomy care.

Chapter 13
The Extra-ocular Muscles

Introduction

There are six extra-ocular muscles which move the eye in the directions of gaze. There are four rectus muscles and two oblique muscles (Fig. 13.1).

- The superior rectus muscle:
  - Origin – the annulus of Zinn, a tendonous ring situated around the apex of the orbit
  - insertion – superior sclera 7.5 mm from the limbus
  - nerve supply – oculomotor nerve
  - primary action – to elevate the eye
  - secondary action – adduction and intorsion.
- The inferior rectus muscle:
  - Origin – the annulus of Zinn
  - insertion – inferior sclera 6.5 mm from the limbus
  - nerve supply – oculomotor nerve
  - primary action – to depress the eye
  - secondary action – adduction and intorsion.
- The medial rectus muscle:
  - Origin – the annulus of Zinn
  - insertion – medial sclera 5.5 mm from the limbus
  - nerve supply – oculomotor nerve
  - primary action – to adduct the eye
  - secondary action – none.
- The lateral rectus muscle:
  - Origin – the annulus of Zinn
  - insertion – lateral sclera 7 mm from the limbus
  - nerve supply – abducens nerve
  - primary action – to abduct the eye
  - secondary action – none.
- The superior oblique muscle:
  - Origin – the annulus of Zinn
  - insertion – superior outer sclera, having passed through the trochlea, a small 'pulley' situated on the medial aspect of the frontal bone (Fig. 13.1); the superior oblique muscle lies inferior to the superior rectus muscle

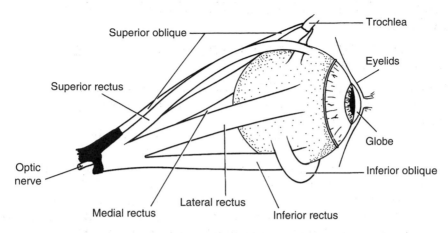

Fig. 13.1 Diagram to show the position of the extra-ocular muscles.

- nerve supply – trochlear nerve
- primary action – to depress the eye
- secondary action – abduction.
- The inferior oblique muscle:
  - Origin – the medial aspect of the maxillary bone
  - insertion – posterior lateral sclera lying inferior to rectus muscle
  - nerve supply – oculomotor nerve
  - primary action – extorsion of the eye
  - secondary action – elevation and abduction.

Note that the primary muscle action relates to the main movement when the eye is in the primary position whilst the secondary action relates to any additional movements the muscle makes to the eye.

Blood supply

Muscular branches of the ophthalmic artery and vein are responsible for supply and drainage of blood.

Eye movements

Both eyes must move together in a co-ordinated manner. In order for this to occur each extra-ocular muscle is paired with a muscle in the opposite eye. These pairs of muscles are known as synergistic or 'yoke' muscles. For example, to look to the right, the right eye looks outwards, i.e. abducts, while the left eye looks inwards, i.e. adducts. The right lateral rectus muscle abducts the right eye, while the left medial rectus muscle adducts the left eye. These two muscles work together to cause the eyes to look to the right.

The right lateral rectus muscle and the left medial rectus muscle are therefore yoke muscles.

Nine positions of gaze

To look directly upwards and downwards, two pairs of yoke muscles are
required to contract. In the other positions, only one pair of yoke muscles is
needed.

The nine positions of gaze, and yoke muscles needed are:

(1)   Straight ahead: the primary position of gaze when all the muscles are
contracting to maintain the eye in this position.
(2)   Upwards to the right: right superior rectus; left inferior oblique.
(3)   To the right: right lateral rectus; left medial rectus.
(4)   Downwards to the right: right inferior rectus; left superior oblique.
(5)   Downwards to the left: left inferior rectus; right superior oblique.
(6)   To the left: left lateral rectus; right medial rectus.
(7)   Upwards to the left: left superior rectus; right inferior oblique.
(8)   Direct elevation: right superior rectus; left inferior oblique *and* left
superior rectus; right inferior oblique.
(9)   Direct depression: right inferior rectus; left superior oblique *and* left
inferior rectus; right superior oblique.

Convergence is the position of the eyes when looking at something close.
In this case both medial recti contract to turn the eye inwards.

Antagonist muscles

When each muscle in the eye contracts, in order for the eye to move the
antagonist or opposite muscle in the same eye must relax to allow the first
muscle to work; for example, to look to the right, the right lateral rectus contracts and the right medial rectus must relax. In the left eye, the left medial
rectus contracts while the left lateral rectus relaxes.

The antagonist muscles are:

• Medial rectus and lateral rectus
• inferior rectus and superior rectus
• inferior oblique and superior oblique.

Strabismus or squint

Strabismus or squint is a deviation of one or either eye in an inward,
outward, upward or downward direction (Fig. 13.2). There are many types
of squint. Only the most common will be described here. Orthoptists are
highly trained to diagnose which muscle is involved and to treat the deviation in conjunction with ophthalmologists.

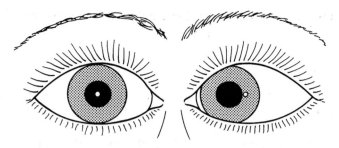

Fig. 13.2 Left convergent squint.

A squint causes diplopia. In a child under eight years of age, this double vision can be suppressed but an adult is unable to do this so the diplopia persists. The child suppresses the vision in the squinting eye so he no longer sees double, which is more comfortable for him. Until the age of eight, the visual process has not matured and if an eye is not used for any reason it may lose its ability to see. This results in reduced visual acuity, a condition called amblyopia. Because the visual system is not mature until the age of eight, reduced vision can be improved with treatment up to this age. Thereafter loss of visual acuity due to amblyopia will not improve. Therefore it is important that squint and any resulting amblyopia are diagnosed before the age of eight years. This applies to all squints, whether manifest or latent. School eye tests are important to pick up poor vision before it is too late for treatment to be of help.

Normal vision with both eyes in use is termed binocular single vision. The images from both eyes together are seen as one visual impression by means of the fusion faculty. The aim of treatment for squint is to restore binocular single vision and prevent or reverse amblyopia.

Squints are either non-paralytic or paralytic.

Non-paralytic squint

Non-paralytic squint is the squint of childhood and is sometimes called a concomitant squint. It can be manifest or latent, convergent or divergent, alternating or non-alternating (unilateral):

- A manifest squint is where one or other eye deviates from the primary or straight ahead position. It can often be an obvious squint to the observer.
- A latent squint is where there is a tendency for both eyes to deviate and this is not usually observed unless symptoms such as headaches or diplopia have occurred, in which case the latent squint may have become manifest.
- A convergent squint is a squint in which one eye turns inwards.
- A divergent squint is a squint in which one eye turns outwards.

- An alternating squint is a squint in which the eyes deviate alternately, whereas it is always the same eye which deviates in a non-alternating squint.

Causes

A non-paralytic squint occurs because there may be obstacles to the correct formation of the image falling on one retina. In other words, there is an obstruction to clear vision in the visual media which results in loss of binocular single vision.

Uncorrected refractive error

Uncorrected refractive error is the commonest cause of squint in childhood. The most usual squint is convergent, the commonest cause being hypermetropia, which causes over-accommodation and therefore over-convergence. In contrast to this, myopia can predispose to a tendency to divergence, because the eyes are already in focus to near vision without the aid of accommodation, convergence is not stimulated and divergence may result. Anisometropia (a different refraction in each eye) causes unequally clear images, which can lead to a squint.

The usual pattern of events to occur (if the onset of squint is under the age of eight years) is:

- squint leads to loss of binocular single vision
- loss of binocular single vision results in diplopia
- diplopia is overcome by suppression of one image
- suppression leads to amblyopia (a reduction in visual acuity in one eye)
- the passage of time leads to loss of binocular function (the two eyes being no longer able to see one image together).

Amblyopia does not develop in an alternating squint as both eyes are used alternatively.

Prolonged eye inactivity

Prolonged inactivity of one eye may be a dissociating factor and may enable the affected eye to deviate through disuse:

- Opacities in the media, i.e. cornea, lens, vitreous or retina, may cause squint. A cataract or retinoblastoma may present as a squint.
- Bandaging of one eye – for example following injury to the eye or a unilateral ptosis – may also cause squint.

Examination

History

A careful history must be taken and should include:

- family history because there may be a hereditary factor
- age at onset which is an important factor in prognosis for reversing amblyopia and restoring binocular single vision
- nature of onset – the onset of squint may occur in one or several of the following ways:
  - suddenly – the squint occurs without any previous sign
  - gradually – the squint appears more and more frequently and possibly increasing in size over a period of time
  - intermittently, e.g. when tired, upset or unwell; the eye may be straight at other times
  - constantly – the squint is present all the time
  - changing in size at different times of day
  - when looking in a particular position of gaze or at a particular distance
  - either eye may deviate alternatively or it may always be the same eye that deviates.

The onset may be associated with some systemic disease because the child is generally unwell.

Visual acuity

Visual acuity will be recorded using the Snellen chart, Sheridan Gardiner test or other tests. Selection of test will be determined by the age, intellectual ability of the patient and their language.

Determination of refractive error

In children a cycloplegic drop such as G. Cyclopentolate 0.5%, by prescription or PGD, is needed to prevent accommodation, which would give a false result on retinoscopy. A retinoscope directs a light beam onto the retina and movement of the retinoscope produces movement of the light beam across the retina in a particular direction. A lens is selected and held in front of the eye while continuing to move the retinoscope. A change is noted in the amount and direction of the movement of the light beam. Finally, the lens, which actually neutralises or abolishes the movement of the light beam, determines the refractive error.

Physical examination

(1) The presence of the following features is noted:
  - epicanthus – if a child has broad epicanthic folds, it can give the

appearance of a convergent squint but if the cover test is negative
this is called a pseudo-squint
  o ptosis or other feature leading to asymmetry of the palpebral
     apertures
  o nystagmus
  o an abnormal head posture, which could be compensating for squint
  o unequal pupil sizes.
(2) An inspection of the eyes is carried out:
  o corneal reflections
  o cover test
  o ocular movements
  o measuring the angle of deviation
  o stereoscopic vision.

The photoscreener has been developed to detect squint, refractive errors
and media opacities in young children without cyclopegia (Ottar et al., 1995).

Corneal reflections

Method

A pen torch is held at $\frac{1}{3}$ m directly in front of both eyes. The position of the
reflection on each eye is then compared.

Results

The results may be:

- normal corneal reflections – symmetrical (Fig. 13.3);
- asymmetrical corneal reflections (Fig. 13.4).

An upturning eye or a down-turning eye can also be detected by observing the corneal reflections (such squints are less common).

Cover test

The cover test is carried out to detect the presence of a squint, and should
be used in conjunction with observation of the corneal reflections.

Method

A penlight is held approximately $\frac{1}{3}$ m from the child. The child must be
looking at the light whilst the cover test is carried out. It is important to
repeat the cover test using a detailed target, e.g. a small picture on a tongue
depressor, because some squints are only present when looking at detailed
objects. The cover test should also be carried out at 6 m where possible
because other squints are only present when looking into the distance, i.e.
intermittent squints.

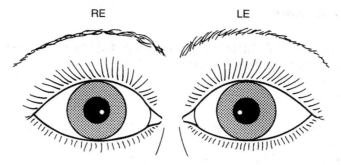

The corneal reflections are symmetrical, usually slightly nasal in each eye.

Note: corneal reflections may not be central, but check **symmetry**.

Fig. 13.3 Normal corneal reflections – symmetrical.

(a)

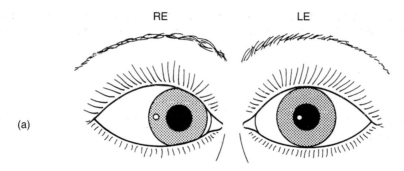

Note asymmetry of corneal reflections.

The left corneal reflection is in the normal position, i.e. slightly nasal.

The right corneal reflection is displaced temporally, because the right eye is turning inwards.

(b)

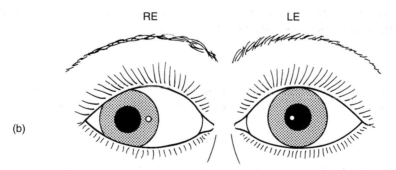

Note asymmetry of corneal reflections.

The left corneal reflection is in the normal position, i.e. slightly nasal.

The right corneal reflection is displaced nasally, because the right eye is turning outwards.

Fig. 13.4 Asymmetrical corneal reflections. (a) Right convergent squint and (b) right divergent squint.

Cover one eye, watching for any movement of the uncovered eye, remove the cover and repeat covering the other eye and watching for any movement of the uncovered eye.

Results

The results may be:

- no manifest squint (Fig. 13.5)
- manifest squint – right convergent squint (Fig. 13.6)
- manfest squint – right divergent squint (Fig. 13.7).

An intermittent convergent squint may not be present when the child is looking at a light but becomes manifest when focusing on a detailed target. Therefore it is important to check the corneal reflections and to carry out the cover test using a light and a detailed target.

An intermittent divergent squint may not be present for near but becomes manifest in the distance. Therefore it is important to carry out a cover test for near and distance. The cover test for a latent squint, or an alternate cover test, is where the occluder covers one eye then the other. Observation of the eye that has just been covered is noted.

Ocular movements

The examiner sits in front of the patient and using a pen torch, and a toy if appropriate, observes both eyes moving in all eight positions of gaze. This will include up, down, both sides and in all four corners, always returning to the straight ahead or primary position. The patient's head must be held still. Any muscle imbalance, over actions and under actions are then noted.

Measuring the angle of deviation

The angle of deviation can be measured using objective or subjective methods. Objective methods are based on the observer neutralising the patient's deviation as it takes up fixation. Subjective measurements are where the patient tells you the position of each image from each eye on a calibrated scale of some sort.

The following methods include both objective and subjective measurements:

- Prisms and cover test: this is the most commonly used objective method of measuring the angle of a manifest or a latent squint. The measurements are performed at near ($^1/_3$ m), distance (6 m) and occasionally beyond 6 m (far distance). Loose prisms, or a prism bar, are introduced in front of the squinting eye in a manifest squint, or in front of either eye in a latent squint, with the apex of the prism in the direction of the deviation.

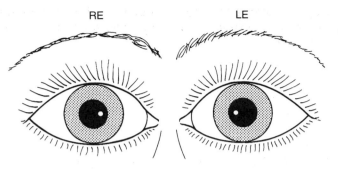

The corneal reflections are symmetrical, i.e. no manifest squint detected.

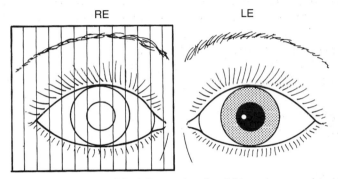

No movement of the left eye when the right eye is covered.

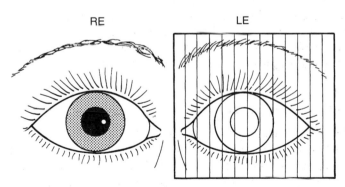

No movement of the right eye when the left eye is covered.

Fig. 13.5 No manifest squint.

- Major amblyoscope (synoptophore): the angle of deviation can be measured both objectively and subjectively. Slides are introduced and the measurement can be read from the scales in degrees or prism dioptres.
- Maddox rod and Maddox wing: The Maddox rod is used in conjunction with a light at 6 m and measures small degrees of squint. The Maddox

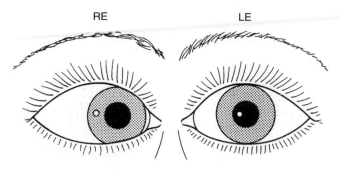

The corneal reflections are asymmetrical, showing a right convergent squint.

Confirm with cover test.

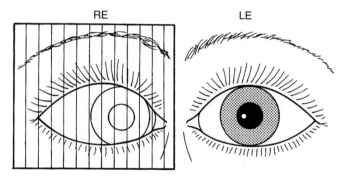

No movement of the left eye when the right eye is covered.

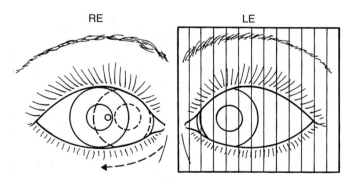

The right eye moves *out* to fix when the left eye is covered.

Fig. 13.6 Manifest squint – right convergent squint.

rod is made of a series of parallel cylinders, red in colour, which convert a light image into a red line. This is placed before one eye while the patient is fixing on a light at 6 m distance with both eyes open. The eye looking through the Maddox rod sees a red line instead of a white light and the other eye sees the light as it really is. These images are too dis-

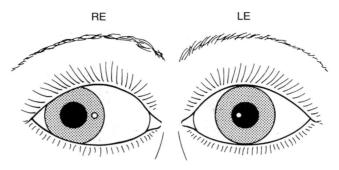

The corneal reflections are asymmetrical, showing a right divergent squint.

Confirm with cover test.

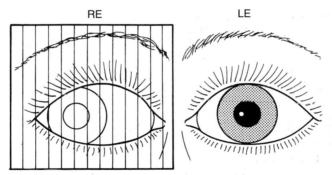

No movement of the left eye when the right eye is covered.

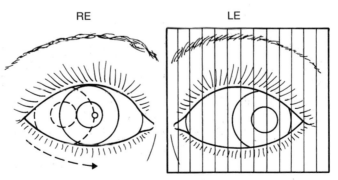

The right eye moves *in* to fix when the left eye is covered.

Fig. 13.7 Manifest squint – right divergent squint.

similar for fusion to take place, so the eyes deviate to the position of squint. Prisms are introduced until the light and the red line are super-imposed. The Maddox wing enables measurements of latent and small manifest deviations to be made at a near distance. The Maddox rod and wing allow measurement of horizontal and vertical deviations. The wing also allows torsional measurements to be made.

Stereoscopic vision

The ability to see in 'depth' or 3D vision is the highest form of binocular sight. The main tests measuring stereo acuity in seconds of arc (the measurement of minimum disparity that gives rise to appreciation of depth) include:

- Frisby test
- Wirt fly test (Titmus test)
- TNO (red/green test)
- Lang stereo test.

See Kanski (2003) for further information.

Treatment

There are several treatment choices for a non-paralytic squint:

- Optical treatment: accurate refraction must be carried out and appropriate glasses ordered. This in itself might correct the squint.
- Occlusion therapy: the visual acuity must be assessed and if amblyopia is present, it must be reversed. This is performed by occluding the 'good' eye to encourage the amblyopic eye to work. Occlusion therapy is carried out, according to the state of amblyopia, in the following ways:
  - total occlusion – the patch is placed over the 'good' eye itself
  - partial occlusion – the lens of the glasses is covered with tape or paper
  - constant occlusion – total or partial occlusion used from morning till night
  - part-time occlusion – total or partial occlusion used for a specified number of hours each day.
- Orthoptic exercises are used to stimulate binocular single vision and strengthen fusion by means of binocular instruments such as the synoptophore. This instrument uses pairs of slides, one for each eye, which match together to form a picture; a bird seen with one eye and a cage seen with the other will be seen with both eyes together as a bird in a cage.
- Operative measures:
  - Early surgery is performed if there is either potential binocular function present; or poor cosmetic appearance with no binocular vision.
  - Surgery can be delayed if the deviation is cosmetically quite good.
  - Surgery is not performed if the cosmetic appearance is good in the presence of no binocular function.

Surgery will not improve binocular vision once it has been lost. The muscles operated on in convergent and divergent squint are usually the medial and lateral recti. They may be resected (shortened) or recessed (effectively lengthened). Sometimes surgery is directed to the non-squinting eye, which worries parents and sometimes nurses! It may not matter which eye is operated on, the aim being to align one eye with the other.

- Botulinum toxin: botulinum toxin (BT) is used to correct some types of convergent and divergent squint, particularly where surgery may be contraindicated as with Graves' disease. It is primarily used for cosmetic reasons. The BT is injected directly into the muscle; however, the paralysis of the muscle is not instantaneous. It can take up to 48 hours to take effect and the action is relatively short lived, between five and eight weeks. Because of this, the treatment needs to be repeated every two to three months.

Paralytic squint

A paralytic or incomitant (non-concomitant) squint is more common in adults than in children. If it occurs in a child under the age of eight years, the child will be able to suppress the resulting double vision and the events that occur with a non-paralytic squint will follow.

Adults, however, have no capacity to suppress the vision in one eye to eliminate the diplopia. This can be distressing and can be associated with nausea and giddiness.

Causes

A paralytic squint is caused by an abnormality in the extra-ocular muscles or their nerve supply.

Muscle disorders

- Trauma, e.g. forceps delivery at birth.
- Congenital abnormality.
- Disease, e.g. exophthalmic ophthalmoplegia from:
  - thyroid eye disease
  - myasthenia gravis
  - neoplasm.

Nerve disorders

Trauma

- Bruising or severing of nerves following head injury.
- Pressure on nerves from haemorrhage.
- Septic infection.

Inflammation

- mastoid disease
- peripheral neuritis
- encephalitis
- multiple sclerosis
- tertiary syphilis
- haemorrhage
- thrombosis
- aneurysm
- neoplasm, e.g. pituitary tumour
- diabetes mellitus
- temporarily following cataract extraction.

Treatment

- Orthoptic assessment to establish which muscle is affected, e.g. examination of eye movements, the Hess chart and diplopia tests.
- Referral to a neurologist or physician for investigation of the cause.
- Teach compensatory head posture, if this is applicable. The patient is taught to hold his head in the position that relieves the diplopia.
- Occlude one eye if the diplopia is intolerable.
- Give temporary Fresnel prism to join the diplopia to binocular single vision if possible.
- Botulinum toxin can be used to paralyse muscles and thereby straighten the eye. It is used to treat strabismus, paralytic strabismus and diplopia post-retinal detachment surgery. Patients need to be aware that the maximum effect is not immediate, but some two to five days later. The effect is only temporary and lasts for between two and three months.
- Wait six to nine months for recovery to occur.
- If recovery does not occur after nine months, surgery can be performed to restore binocular single vision.

Patient's needs (non-paralytic and paralytic squint)

- Correction of squint for cosmetic reasons (children are especially teased at school).
- Correction of amblyopia and restoration of binocular single vision.
- Relief of diplopia if an adult.

Nursing action (non-paralytic and paralytic squint)

- Assist with examination in the outpatient department.
- Instil prescribed cycloplegic drops, e.g. G. Cyclopentolate hydrochloride.
- Liaise with the orthoptic department if necessary about patching and exercises, and offer teaching and encouragement to the parents and child on the use of patching.

- Give advice on occluding one eye, prisms in glasses or compensatory head posture to relieve the symptoms.
- Prepare the patient for botulinum injections.
- Admit the patient to day unit if surgery is to be performed.
- Give pre-operative care, e.g. explain reasons for possibility of surgeon operating on the 'good' eye. Warn adult patients that they may feel unwell for about a week; the reason for this is not readily understood.
- Give post-operative care:
  - The eye is not usually padded post-operatively.
  - There may be conjunctival injection present, including a subconjunctival haemorrhage.
  - Instil prescribed antibiotic or steroid and antibiotic drops.
  - Give analgesia intramuscularly if adjustable sutures have been employed prior to their being adjusted. This can occur any time from immediately coming round from the anaesthetic to 24 hours later. Adjustable sutures are suitable for any patient over the age of ten (Pratt-Johnson & Tillson, 1994). Topical anaesthetic is used immediately prior to adjustment such as G. Oxybuprocaine 0.4% to facilitate adjustment.
  - Liaise with the orthoptic department regarding the necessity of continuing with non-surgical treatment such as wearing glasses, occlusion, etc.
  - Avoid swimming, contact sports for four weeks.
  - Children should only need to be kept off school for a few days.
- Ensure that the patient has a follow-up orthoptic appointment on discharge.

Complications (non-paralytic and paralytic squint)

- Stitch abscess.
- The muscle slipping away from its new position because the sutures have broken.
- Failure of the operation to result in binocular single vision when this is the expected outcome.
- Failure of the operation to give a good cosmetic result.
- Overcorrection of the squint. A convergent squint results in a consecutive divergent squint, and vice versa.

Pseudosquint

A pseudosquint is the appearance of a squint occurring in the presence of binocular single vision.

Causes

- Epicanthus.
- Abnormal angle alpha: this is a larger or smaller than normal angle between the optic axis and the visual axis. This angle is very similar to that of angles kappa and gamma.
- Facial asymmetry.
- Wide or narrow interpupillary distance: a wide interpupillary distance gives the appearance of divergent squint; and a narrow interpupillary distance, convergent squint.

Chapter 14
Ophthalmic Trauma

Introduction

The ophthalmic nurse requires special skills of observation (see Chapter 3), history-taking and the ability to care for a patient who has received trauma to the eye or its surrounding area (see Chapter 2).

Penetrating (perforating) injury and ocular burns are considered ophthalmic emergencies. Blunt trauma can result in serious ocular damage. Therefore the nurse must take an accurate history, examine the eye carefully and decide in what order of priority each patient presenting with ocular trauma needs to be placed.

A blow to the eyeball causes shock waves to pass through it, damaging many structures such as the cornea, iris, lens and retina. Blunt trauma may accompany a penetrating injury, therefore any patient presenting with a history of a forceful blow to the eye must have all ocular structures examined carefully. The importance of accurate history-taking and accurate measurement of visual acuity cannot be overemphasised.

Children presenting with ocular trauma whose history is not appropriate for the injury sustained must be carefully screened for any sign of child abuse and appropriate action taken if found.

Minims drops which are sterile and preservative free must be used in all eye examination for ocular trauma.

Patients presenting with ocular trauma must have their visual acuity checked to establish baseline reading.

It is assumed in the following text that all patients will be treated for accompanying shock if present and that this may be a priority. Where appropriate a tetanus toxoid injection must be given if the skin or ocular tissue has been cut.

Intra-ocular foreign body

An intra-ocular foreign body (IOFB) results when something enters the eye under force, such as fragments generated when using a hammer and chisel or a lathe. The foreign body may lodge itself in any of the structures of the eye and examination may not reveal its presence, highlighting the importance of history-taking. History-taking should include whether appropriate eye protection has been worn at time of injury.

Patient's needs

- Thorough ocular examination to determine the extent of the injuries.
- Explanation of the extent of the injuries and the required treatment.
- Admission to hospital for removal of the IOFB.
- Post-operative and discharge care.

Nursing action

- Obtain accurate history.
- Inform medical staff.
- Prepare the patient for an X-ray or CT scan to locate the IOFB.
- Prepare the patient for removal of the foreign body if one is present. If it is metallic, it may be removed with a specialised magnet in the operating theatre.
- Give post-operative care, clean the eye, instill drops. Give any necessary information including advice on appropriate eye protection to prevent future injuries.
- Plan discharge.

Fracture of the orbit

Fractures of the orbit occur as a result of trauma. Usually they are easily recognised by the irregularity of the outline of the orbit. A 'blow-out' fracture of the orbit occurs following trauma to the maxillary bone which fractures and the eye tends to sink down into the gap created in the bone. Patients with suspected 'blow-out' fracture should be told not to blow their nose to minimise emphysema. Emphysema (the skin crackles when pressed) may be present due to a fracture maxillary sinus.

Signs and symptoms

- Enophthalmos.
- Inability to move the eye in all fields of gaze because the extra-ocular muscles have become trapped in the fractured bone.
- Jerky eye movement in the upward gaze because the inferior oblique and inferior rectus muscle have been trapped.
- Diplopia.
- Areas of facial paraesthesia which may suggest damage of the infra-orbital or supra-orbital nerve damage.

Patient's needs

- Diagnosis of the presence of a fracture.
- Relief of symptoms of:
  - decreased sensation of the skin over the maxilla
  - diplopia.

- Repair of skin laceration if present.
- Repair of fracture if severe (may not be performed for up to six months).
- Cleaning of any wounds present.

Nursing action

- Explain to the patient the extent of the injuries and the treatment to be carried out.
- Preparation for X-ray examination to confirm and isolate the fracture.
- Clean wound if present.
- Admit the patient to the ward if surgery is to be performed.
- Prepare the patient for the operation to free the trapped muscles and repair the fracture. A Teflon plate or orbital implant may be inserted.
- Give post-operative care:
  - clean the wound
  - instil antibiotic drops
  - give prescribed systemic antibiotics.
- Plan discharge.
- Remove sutures, usually as an outpatient procedure, five to seven days post-operatively.

Trauma to the eyelids

Trauma to the eyelids is a common occurrence as their function is to protect the globe. The following may occur:

- bruising
- laceration
- burns.

Patient's needs

- Exploration of the extent of the injuries.
- Relief of symptoms: if a subtarsal foreign body is present there will be profuse lacrimation and blepharospasm.
- Treatment of injuries.

Nursing priorities

- Inform medical staff.
- Commence irrigation if a burn has occurred.

Nursing action

- Explain to the patient the extent of the injuries received and the necessary treatment.
- Assist the doctor in examining the eye.

- Treat the injuries:
  - Bruising: apply cold compress and instruct the patient how to do this.
  - Laceration:
    - (i)   Clean wound.
    - (ii)   Prepare the patient and equipment for suturing of the laceration or apply Steristrip if superficial. The two edges of the lacerated lid must be aligned very carefully to prevent trichiasis occurring.
  - Burns:
    - (i)   Clean area.
    - (ii)   Irrigate eye (see p. 39).
    - (iii) Admit patient if necessary.
    - (iv)   Do not pad an eye with an ocular burn.
    - (v)   Prepare the patient for skin grafting which may need to be carried out before scar tissue forms.
  - Subtarsal foreign body: remove the foreign body (see p. 36).

Trauma to the lacrimal system

Laceration of the lacrimal drainage apparatus is fairly common. If the canaliculus is torn accurate apposition of the tear ducts must be performed to prevent permanent epiphora. In children the injury is often caused by the claws of a dog as it jumps up to greet the child.

Patient's needs

- Cleaning of the wound.
- Admission to hospital if necessary.
- Repair of the laceration.
- Prophylactic antibiotic cover.
- Analgesia as required.

Nursing priorities

- Inform medical staff of the extent of the injuries.

Nursing action

- Clean the wound.
- Assist the doctor to examine the wound.
- Admit the patient to the ward if necessary.
- Prepare the patient for surgery to repair the laceration.
- Give post-operative care:
  - clean the wound
  - instil antibiotic drops
  - analgesia as required
  - give oral antibiotics if prescribed
  - remove sutures five to seven days post-operatively.

Trauma to the conjunctiva

Subconjunctival haemorrhage

Subconjunctival haemorrhage (Fig. 14.1) can result from a penetrating or blunt trauma which causes the conjunctival blood vessels to bleed.

Patient's needs

- Investigation into the extent of the injuries.

Nursing action

- Obtain accurate history.
- Examine the patient or assist the doctor. It is important to be able to visualise the scleral margin posterior to the bleed. If it is absent the bleeding may have tracked from elsewhere, typically the anterior cranial fossa, and is more serious.
- Reassure the patient that the haemorrhage will not cover the cornea and so not affect vision.
- Inform the patient that the blood may spread before it resolves and that it may take two to three weeks to clear completely, similar to a bruise. There is no specific treatment for the haemorrhage.

Laceration of the conjunctiva

Laceration of the conjunctiva may occur as a result of trauma to the eye. The eye must be examined to see if the underlying sclera has been involved. If there is a possibility of a foreign body having entered the eye, an X-ray must be taken to exclude or confirm this.

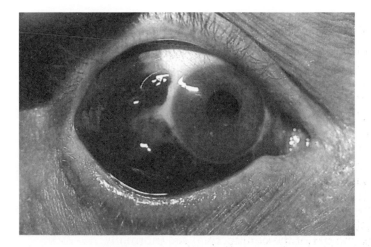

Fig. 14.1 Subconjunctival haemorrhage.

Patient's needs

- Cleaning and examination of the wound and eye to discover the extent of the injuries.
- Suturing of the wound if necessary. This is not always performed.
- Prophylactic antibiotic cover.

Nursing action

- Inform the doctor of the patient's condition.
- Assist the doctor in the examination.
- Prepare the patient and equipment for cleaning and suturing of the laceration under local anaesthetic, unless the patient is a child, when a general anaesthetic will usually be administered. Small lacerations may be left to heal without suturing.
- Apply pad following the procedure.

Ocular burns

Ocular burns can result in patients losing their sight.

Acid substances entering the eye coagulate with the protein of the ocular surface and cease to act although damage is caused by the initial impact. Alkaline substances, such as lime found in cement and brick dust, continue to be active in the eye, destroying the superficial layers and penetrating the anterior segment of the eye. Collagenase is released by the cornea following an alkali burn and this destroys the cornea. It is therefore vitally important that the eye(s) are thoroughly cleaned of all particles of lime. Immediate washing of the eye with whatever harmless liquid is at hand is the best first aim measure that can be employed. The patient should then be transferred to an ophthalmic unit. The eye must never be padded following chemical injury.

Patient's needs

- Irrigation of eye(s).
- Treatment of burns to the lids and skin around the eye that may have occurred.
- Reassurance and information on the extent of the injuries and treatment. Patients can be very worried about the threat of sight loss following a chemical burn.
- Pain relief.

Nursing priorities

- If a severe alkali burn has occurred, inform the doctor immediately of the patient's arrival.
- Check the pH of the conjunctival sac (normally 7.3–7.7).

- Commence irrigation of the eye(s) after instillation of local anaesthetic drop (see p. 39). If working single-handed, commence the irrigation before informing the doctor.

Nursing action

- Irrigate the eye(s) (see p. 39). Ensure all particles have been removed. It may be necessary to double evert the lid.
- Allay anxiety.
- Test visual acuity once the patient's condition allows you to.
- Institute the following treatment which will be prescribed after the eye has been examined to establish the extent of the damage to the conjunctiva and the cornea.

Mild burns

- Instil G. Homatropine 2% to 'rest' the eye and prevent uveitis.
- Instil G. or Oc. Chloramphenicol to prevent infection and provide lubrication.
- Give prescribed analgesia.

Moderate to severe burns (Fig. 14.2)

This level of burn is illustrated in Fig. 14.2.

- Instil:
  - potassium ascorbate drops to aid healing, intensively such as hourly initially, reducing to two-hourly after three days; advise the patient that these drops sting
  - G. Chloramphenicol to prevent infection
  - a steroid such as G. Dexamethasone (maxidex) to prevent/treat inflammation

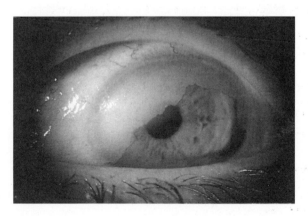

Fig. 14.2 Lime burn.

- ○ G. Homatropine 2% to 'rest' the eye and prevent/treat uveitis.
- Drugs that inhibit collagenase such as metaloproteinase inhibitors may be used.
- Apply a bandage contact lens to prevent symblephron forming. Rodding of the fornices may be employed.
- Apply steroid ointment to the skin around the eye if prescribed.

Other treatments

The excimer laser has been used to treat chemical burns. Keratoepithelioplasty (KEP) or cadaveric limbal cell transplantation has also been successfully employed.

Complications

Symblephron

Symblephron is the adhesion of the bulbar conjunctiva to the palpebral conjunctiva (Fig. 14.3). It occurs following alkaline burns to the eye when the epithelial layer of the conjunctiva is stripped off and the two areas of the conjunctiva stick together. When this occurs the fornices are lost and the eye is immobile. The lids may not be able to cover and protect the eyeball. It is therefore important to keep the fornices well lubricated and to apply a bandage contact lens to separate the two conjunctival surfaces or to rod them to break up any adhesions that might occur. This latter procedure can be painful. Nasal mucosal grafts can be performed.

Corneal opacities

Corneal opacities occur from destruction of the layers of the cornea from the burns. Blindness may result.

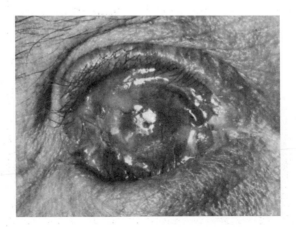

Fig. 14.3 Symblephron.

Welder's flash

Welder's flash or a burn from a sun lamp or snowblindness burn the cornea if protective goggles have not been worn. Both eyes are affected and become very red and sore typically after six hours.

Patient's needs

- Relief of symptoms of: acute pain; watering; photophobia; and reduced vision.

These symptoms do not become evident until about eight hours after the incident has occurred.

Nursing action

- Instil local anaesthetic drops. Local anaesthetic drops must never be given to patient to take home as these drops inhibit epithelial healing.
- Institute prescribed treatment once the eye has been examined. G. fluorescein shows punctate staining over most of the cornea, especially within a central band. The treatment is with:
  - ○ Oc. Chloramphenicol immediately – once only
  - ○ pad and bandage if severe; both eyes may need to be bandaged for comfort and healing.

Trauma to the cornea

Corneal foreign bodies

Many different kinds of foreign bodies can adhere to the cornea: dirt specks, sawdust, pieces of metal or rust (Fig. 14.4). Anyone working in an environment, whether at work or at home, where particles can fly into the eye, or working with a hammer and chisel, should wear protective goggles. But these do not always afford complete protection.

The eye with a corneal foreign body present may or may not be red, depending on what the foreign body is, how long it has been in the eye and how much the patient has rubbed it.

Patient's needs

- Removal of the foreign body to relieve pain and discomfort.
- Treatment of any corneal abrasion.

Nursing action

- Record the visual acuity before removal of the foreign body. This is particularly important if the accident has occurred at work. It may be

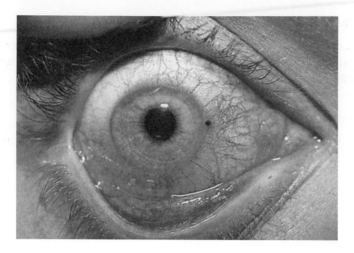

Fig. 14.4 Metallic corneal foreign body.

necessary to instil a drop of local anaesthetic into the eye before the patient can read the Snellen chart.
- Assist the doctor or nurse practitioner to remove the foreign body (see p. 36).
- Apply antibiotic ointment.
- Apply a pad if necessary for patient comfort but bear in mind recent research indicating that the corneal epithelium is slower to heal under a pad (Visto, 2000)
- If the foreign body is a piece of metal, a rust ring may be left around the abrasion resulting from the foreign body. This rust ring will need to be removed either at the first visit or the following one. A dental burr may be used for this procedure.
- Instil G. Homatropine 2% to prevent the complication of uveitis occurring.
- Ensure the patient is not driving if he has an eye pad on. Although it is not illegal to drive with one eye padded, it is not safe to do so and the patient's insurance will not be valid. Stereoscopic vision is lost and the field of vision reduced, especially if the right eye is covered. If the patient has arrived by car and there is no-one to take him home, he can be given a pad to apply at home following instructions on how to do so.
- Ensure the patient understands the need for any follow-up visit(s) required to check on healing.

Complications
- Corneal ulceration.
- Corneal scarring.

Corneal abrasion

Corneal abrasions can result from a foreign body as seen above. Other common causes are babies' fingernails, twigs, flower stalks, pens and pencils. In fact a great variety of items can cause abrasion.

Patient's needs

- Relief of symptoms, which can vary in severity: pain; lacrimation; photophobia; blepharospasm; and reduced vision.
- Treatment of the abrasion.

Nursing action

- Record visual acuity. It may be necessary to instil a local anaesthetic drop first.
- Examine/assist the doctor to examine the eye. The abraded area will show up with the instillation of G. Fluorescein and illumination with a blue light.
- Institute prescribed treatment:
  - If large, G. Homatropine 2% will be instilled to prevent uveitis and afford some pain relief as the pupil will dilate and prevent iris spasm.
  - Apply Oc. Chloramphenicol.
  - Apply a pad or pad and bandage if the abrasion is large (see p. 32).
- Warn the patient that this condition will be painful and ensure he has adequate analgesia to take.
- Short term non-steroidal anti-inflammatory such as Voltarol may be prescribed as a topical analgesia for pain management. Long term use of Voltarol is not advocated due to the likelihood of corneal melt. Caution should be exercised when prescribing any non-steroidal anti-inflammatory in the presence of any underlying corneal pathology such as a history of herpes virus infection or keratocconus.
- Ensure the patient understands the need for any follow-up visit(s) required to check on healing. A large abrasion may take several days to heal.

Complications

- Corneal ulceration.
- Recurrent corneal abrasion/erosion: these can recur up to one year or longer after the initial incident. The patient on waking finds he has difficulty opening the eye and that it is painful. On examination the epithelium will have debrided again. This occurs because the epithelium is loosely adherent to Bowman's membrane. There may be an hereditary tendency to recurrent erosions. The treatment is as above. The excimer laser has been used to treat these erosions. Application of eye ointment such as simple eye ointment at night can prevent this recurring condition.

Perforation of the cornea

Usually when the cornea perforates from injury, the iris herniates into the perforation, blocking it and causing the anterior chamber to collapse (Fig. 14.5).

Patient's needs

- Immediate attention.
- Relief of anxiety about possible loss of the eye.
- Admission to hospital.

Nursing priorities

- Inform medical staff of the patient's injuries.

Nursing action

- Allay anxiety.
- Record visual acuity if possible.
- Assist the doctor to examine the eye.
- Clean any wounds around the eye.
- Admit the patient to hospital for:
  - rest and recovery from the accident
  - pre-operative care prior to excision of prolapsed iris, repair of corneal wound and restoration of anterior chamber; if the prolapsed iris shows no signs of deterioration and has not been prolapsed for long, it may be repositioned under intensive antibiotic cover.
- Post-operative care. Observe the eye for:
  - hyphaema
  - depth of anterior chamber.

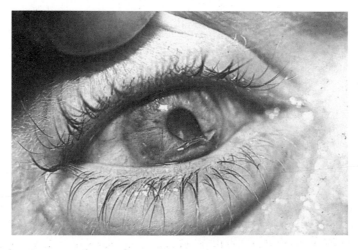

Fig. 14.5 Perforating corneal wound.

Complications

Immediate

- Loss of anterior chamber.
- Disorganisation of ocular contents.
- Endophthalmitis.

Long term

- Corneal scarring.
- Astigmatism due to scarring.
- Glaucoma.
- Recurrent uveitis.
- Phthisis bulbi.

Trauma of the uveal tract

Hyphaema

Following blunt or penetrating injury to the uveal tract, the iris or ciliary body may bleed into the anterior chamber causing a hyphaema (see Fig. 14.6 and Colour Plate 4). If, by looking through a slit lamp, the blood cells are seen floating in the anterior chamber, prior to settling inferiorally, this is termed a microscopic hyphaema.

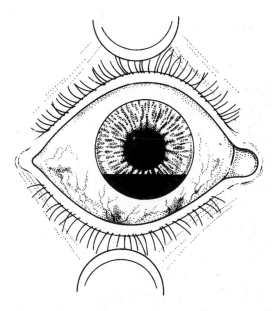

Fig. 14.6 Hyphaema. (Reproduced with permission from Vaughan, D.G. & Asbury, T. (1983) *General Ophthalmology* (10th edn), Appleton & Lange.)

A blackball hyphaema is one which fills the whole of the anterior chamber. Sometimes the blood clots in the anterior chamber and may be attached to the iris.

Patient's needs

Treatment of the hyphaema by:

- rest at home
- admission to hospital.

Nursing action

- Inform medical staff of the patient's condition and history of trauma.
- Admit the patient if necessary.
- Inform the patient of the importance of rest. A severe bleed may occur 48 hours later in a minority of patients, especially if the large ciliary body vessels have bled. The intra-ocular pressure may rise acutely and a prolonged rise in IOP can cause damage to the optic nerve.
- Prepare the patient for an anterior chamber washout in the case of a blackball hyphaema or if the hyphaema has not resolved after four to five days.
- Give post-operative care. Eye care:
  o instil prescribed drops, e.g. G. chloramphenicol and G. maxidex (dexamethasone)
  o observe the anterior chamber for depth and recurrence of hyphaema.
- Following a blow to the eye the fundus needs to be examined. There is differing opinion as to whether this should be carried out immediately. Some authorities believe immediate dilation will induce further bleeding (Ragge & Easty, 1990).

Complications

- Secondary bleed 24–48 hours after the initial injury.
- Secondary glaucoma:
  o the blood cells or clot in the anterior chamber blocks the drainage angle
  o angle recession following trauma, which may not become evident for some years, so the patient must have annual eye examinations.
- In long-standing hyphaema the cornea may become blood-stained.

Traumatic mydriasis

Following trauma (usually blunt) to the iris, the pupil may become fixed and dilated. This is due to paralysis of the sphincter muscle in the iris. It may resolve itself after a few days. If it is permanent, the patient will experience photophobia.

Trauma to the lens

Traumatic cataract

Cataract formation can result from a direct or indirect assault on the lens; for example a penetrating injury, such as a hammer and chisel injury, or a blunt injury, such as from a squash ball. An intra-ocular foreign body may lodge on the lens causing a surrounding opacity. This may be the only indication of the intra-ocular foreign body. Trauma to the lens during intra-ocular surgery falls into this category. When the capsule of the lens is injured, aqueous enters the lens substance, causing it to swell and become cloudy. Opacities are most often found in the posterior cortex and sometimes appear like a flower with several petals. They gradually enlarge to cover the whole lens. Lens matter may leak out of the injured capsule into the anterior chamber, where it may cause uveitis or a secondary (phacolytic) glaucoma by blocking the drainage angle. Leaked lens matter can be absorbed by the aqueous, in which case it will not cause any complications.

The development of a traumatic cataract can occur from within a few hours after the incident to months later.

Treatment of a traumatic cataract is similar to that of other causes (see p. 149).

Trauma to the retina vitreous choroid and optic nerve

Trauma to the posterior segment of the eye may result in a vitreous haemorrhage, retinal tear, retinal detachment (p. 165), choroidal haemorrhage, choroidal tear, macular tear, optic nerve contusion, or commotio retinae (oedema of the retina).

Patient's needs

- Accurate diagnosis and prognosis.
- Preparation for repair of damaged structures (see Vitrectomy and Types of retinal detachment surgery on p. 167).
- Post-operative care and discharge planning.

Nursing action

- Take an accurate history.
- Report to medical staff.
- Assist in examination.
- Allay the patient's anxiety.
- Prepare the patient for surgery as appropriate (see p. 166).
- Give post-operative care (see p. 166).
- Plan discharge.
- Commotio retinae is managed by rest.

Prevention of ocular trauma and eye protection

Nurses working in the ophthalmic casualty area are ideally suited to advise patients on how to prevent ocular trauma. Posters can be displayed in the waiting area and public places outside the hospital that highlight the danger to eyes from certain activities and what protection is available. Eye protection should be worn for racquet sports and for some contact sports as well as in industry. The incidence of ocular trauma has risen with the increase in DIY activities. Suppliers of DIY equipment do not always emphasise the need for eye protection, although hire firms are obliged to. There are many types of eye protectors on the market, although some scratch easily or become steamed up. The most effective protectors are more expensive to purchase.

Chapter 15
Removal of an Eye

Removal of an eye

An eye is removed if it is blind and painful, usually as a result of chronic or secondary glaucoma, if there is severe infection or malignancy, or following severe trauma.

There are three operative procedures for removal of an eye. The decision of the surgeon to opt for a particular method is determined by the nature of the pathology (Jones, 2001).

(1) *Enucleation* This is the surgical removal of the eyeball itself. The extra-ocular muscles and remaining orbital contents are conserved. The muscles are utilised to create movement of the prosthetic eye. It is performed when the eye is blind and painful; following trauma to the globe; or for malignancy which is confined to the globe, such as a malignant choroidal melanoma or retinoblastoma. In cases of malignancy a length of optic nerve must be removed as well to ensure that the disease has not spread along the nerve fibres. If the nerve is found to be involved, radiotherapy will be given to the socket. Cases where the patient has enucleated their own eye, whilst rare, do happen. Such patients usually have underlying psychological or psychiatric problems.

(2) *Evisceration* is the removal of the contents of the globe leaving the sclera intact. This is performed following trauma and in cases of severe infection, the sclera being left in situ to prevent infection spreading into the brain via the optic nerve and ophthalmic blood vessels. The sclera provides scaffolding for any subsequent implant and prosthetic eye.

(3) *Exenteration* is the removal of the total contents of the orbit and if necessary the eyelids, plus any involved bone. This is performed for malignancy that is outside the eyeball, such as a basal cell carcinoma of the eyelid that has eroded structures behind it.

Removal of the eye should never be performed before a second opinion is obtained as to its necessity.

Patient's needs

Some patients will already be in hospital following trauma or infection when the decision to remove the eye is taken. Others will need to be admitted. If the eye is blind and painful, the patient may be relieved at the thought of its removal. Some people, though, resist having the eye removed despite severe pain, preferring to rely on analgesics or nerve blocks for pain relief. It may be worth pointing out to these patients that a blind eye gradually shrinks (phthisis bulbi) and becomes unsightly.

Removal of an eye is an emotive subject and most patients will be highly anxious about the social, physical and psychological effects and will need much support. The patient's reaction to having an eye removed will vary according to his individual personality, family support, age and gender as well as the circumstances surrounding the cause of the removal.

A very young child will not understand fully what is happening and may quickly adapt to a prosthesis as he will have known little else. However, the parents will be feeling very differently, requiring a great amount of support. They may be suffering acute guilt feelings, especially if the child had an accident for which they blame themselves. Siblings and friends may also be upset, especially if they have been involved in, or caused, the accident.

All patients of any age will go through a period of loss for their eye, including feelings of anger and resentment, while coming to terms with their condition. Teenagers may be particularly concerned about their appearance and body image, which may prevent them from socialising with their peers. All age groups and both sexes will be very aware of their changed appearance. They will be much more critical of their prosthesis, noting minute differences to their other eye. It is worth pointing out to them that no two natural eyes in the same face are exactly similar.

Some families and friends will be able to give the patient the necessary support, but others may not feel able to. Some family members may require help from the nurse to come to terms with the patient's loss.

Nursing action

- Admit the patient to hospital.
- Give psychological and practical help. Explain about prostheses (see below) to the patient, pointing out that these days they are very good matches and need not be removed. It may be helpful to put him in touch with a patient who already has a prosthesis. A visit by the prosthetist before the operation will result in the patient having a better understanding of the processes involved in creating the artificial eye. The patient needs to understand that the prosthesis will not be placed in the socket at the time of surgery but at a later stage. In addition they should be advised that post-operatively they will have a dressing of pad and bandage, worn undisturbed for a week. First dressing takes place in the outpatient setting. They should be advised also that it is not unusual to suffer nausea and vomiting immediately post-operatively. They should be reassured that the nurse will give analgesia and anti-emetics as required (Waterman et al., 1998). If the patient is a child, the parents must be totally involved in his care.
- Give pre-operative care.

- Give post-operative care:
  - ○ Remove pressure dressing at the first dressing, clean socket and instil prescribed antibiotic ointment. Subsequently the socket will be cleaned regularly and the ointment instilled. No further dressing is applied.
  - ○ If the socket is clean, fit a temporary shell into it.
  - ○ Teach the patient or parents to remove, clean and replace the shell (see p. 45), and instil antibiotic ointment.
- On discharge, ensure that the patient has an appointment with the prosthetist and give him the assurance that he can return at any time to the hospital if there are any problems with the shell.

Complications

- The socket may become infected at any stage following removal of the eye. This requires cleaning of the socket and antibiotic treatment, usually ointment.
- The socket may shrink with time, causing the prosthesis to protrude and making it appear much larger than the other eye. A new prosthesis will need to be made.

Prostheses

Once the initial socket dressing has been removed following surgery and the socket is clean, a temporary shell is inserted into the socket to maintain the shape of the eyelids, to prevent them retracting. The patient is taught to remove, clean and replace this and make sure the socket is clean.

At four to six weeks following surgery the patient is fitted with a temporary artificial eye by the prosthetist. This may be fitted earlier if the patient's needs warrant it. Initially a temporary prosthesis is fitted which will match as nearly as possible the patient's other eye. Meanwhile a permanent individualised prosthesis will be made from an impression of the socket. The colour of the sclera, the pattern of the conjunctival vessels, the colour and pattern of the iris and the position of the pupil will be painted on by hand, carefully matching the other eye. Prosthetists are perfectionists who pay attention to the smallest of details.

Prostheses are nowadays made of an inert plastic material which can remain in the socket for up to a year. If there are no problems, the prosthesis is cleaned and polished annually to smooth any rough surfaces.

A prosthesis will need to be removed if it becomes too big for the shrinking socket or if the colour of the other eye changes – as it does with age – the sclera becoming less white and the conjunctival blood vessels more pronounced. The iris may change colour and an arcus senilis may appear.

Prostheses are made to measure and with careful matching of the other eye it is often difficult to tell an artificial eye from a real one (Fig. 15.1). Sometimes the movement of the prosthesis is not as good as in a normal eye. Fol-

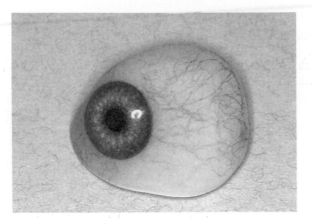

Fig. 15.1 A prosthesis.

lowing an evisceration, movement should be nearly normal as the extra-ocular muscles are still in place and can move the prosthesis. During an enu-cleation the extra-ocular muscles are cut from their insertion in the sclera and sutured together in the socket. This affords some movement of the prosthe-sis. Primary socket implantation can be carried out, whereby an acrylic or coralline hydroxyapatite implant is placed in the socket to which the extra-ocular muscles are attached by sutures. This affords more movement of the prosthesis. Implants can be rejected and they tend to extrude after about 20 years, requiring replacement although the hydroxyapatite type aims to over-come this. Being a naturally-derived material from coral, with a similar struc-ture to bone, it is not rejected by the body. The body tissue actually grows into the implant. A peg can be used to attach the prosthesis to the hydro-xyapatite implant to afford greater movement of the prosthesis when it is in situ (Dutton, 1991). After an exenteration, it is not possible to fit a prosthesis into the socket without further plastic surgery. A prosthesis can be attached to spectacles for patients not wishing to undergo further surgery.

Chapter 16
Ocular Manifestations of Systemic Disease

This chapter summarises the effects of systemic eye disease on the eye. Most of the detailed information has already been discussed and can be found in the chapters on the diseases of the specific ocular structures.

Diabetes mellitus

Diabetes mellitus can cause the following ocular conditions:

- Lids:
    - styes (see p. 72)
    - chalazions (see p. 68).
- Cornea: keratitis (see p. 106).
- Iris:
    - rubeosis iridis from neovascularisation (see p. 144)
    - atrophy of the iris
    - spontaneous hyphaema from rubeosis iridis
- Chronic open-angle glaucoma.
- Secondary glaucoma from rubeosis iridis and peripheral anterior synaechiae (see p. 144).
- Lens:
    - cataract (see p. 152)
    - intermittent refractive errors due to changes in blood glucose levels and therefore changes in the glucose levels in the lens.
- Uveal tract: uveitis (see p. 123).
- Retina:
    - retinal vein occlusion (see p. 170)
    - retinopathy (see p. 172)
    - retinal detachment (see p. 165).

- Vitreous: haemorrhage (see p. 184).

- Optic nerve:
    - retrobulbar neuritis (see p. 183)
    - optic atrophy (see p. 183).

- Nerve palsies: this occurs, rarely, due to inflammation of the third, fourth and sixth cranial nerves causing paralysis of the extra-ocular muscles.

Acquired immune deficiency syndrome (AIDS)

AIDS can cause the following conditions:

- Microvascular disease:
  - retina – usually asymptomatic:
    - (i)   cotton wool spots
    - (ii)   haemorrhages
    - (iii) microaneurysms
  - conjunctiva – vessels have altered appearance.
- Opportunistic infections affecting the retina:
  - cytomegalovirus (CMV) (see p. 178)
  - herpes simplex and zoster
  - toxoplasmosis
  - candida
  - tuberculosis
  - syphilis
  - molluscum contagiosum
  - pneumocystis.
- Neoplasms:
  - Kaposi' s sarcoma:
    - (i)   eyelid
    - (ii)   conjunctiva
    - (iii) nose
    - (iv)   orbit
  - Burkitt's lymphoma: orbit.
- Neuro-ophthalmic:
  - cranial nerve palsies
  - visual field defects
  - papilloedema
  - optic atrophy.

Thyroid disease

Thyrotoxicosis affects the eye in the following ways (see p. 66):

- lid lag
- lid retraction
- exophthalmos
- conjunctival chemosis
- exposure keratitis
- ophthalmoplegia.

Complications

- Corneal ulceration leading to perforation.
- Optic nerve compression.
- Glaucoma.
- Central retinal artery and vein occlusion.
- Cataract.

Hypertension

Hypertension causes a retinopathy (see p. 175).

Giant cell arteritis

Giant cell arteritis or temporal arteritis is a condition of those from the over 60s age group, affecting all arteries, having an effect especially on the heart and kidneys. It is also associated with polymyalgia rheumatica. In the eye it causes a sudden loss of vision in one or both eyes. This is caused by infarctions in the ciliary arteries which supply the optic nerve head causing ischaemia and swelling of the optic disc. The temporal artery is often prominent, hard and tender to touch.

Patient's needs

- Relief of symptoms:
  - sudden loss of vision
  - general malaise
  - temporal headaches
  - pain on chewing
  - tenderness on scalp when combing hair.
- Institution of treatment.

Nursing priority

Inform the doctor of the patient's history of sudden loss of vision.

Nursing action

- Instil prescribed mydriatic drops to facilitate ophthalmoscopy.
- Assist the doctor to take blood for ESR estimation. A high reading is indicative of giant cell arteritis. It can be as high as 100 mmHg in one hour.
- Prepare patient and equipment and assist the doctor in performing a temporal artery biopsy. This is not always performed as a false negative result can occur.

- Admit the patient to hospital if the condition is severe enough to warrant high-dose systemic steroids, maybe via the intravenous route.
- If the patient is not admitted, explain the treatment by oral steroids and the importance of carrying a steroid card.
- Ensure the patient has an outpatient follow-up appointment.
- High doses of oral steroids are given to prevent further visual loss in the presenting eye if unilateral and to prevent the disease affecting the other eye. These steroids will be gradually reduced and the disease monitored by regular ESR estimations. A maintenance dose of steroids may need to be continued for several years. Patients with severe visual loss resulting from this disease may need to be registered as blind or partially sighted (see p. 2).

Herpes simplex virus

Herpes simplex virus causes a conjunctivitis and keratitis resulting in a dendritic corneal ulcer (see p. 108).

Herpes zoster virus

In the eye the herpes zoster virus affects the trigeminal nerve (see p. 109). Usually only the ophthalmic branch is involved, but the maxillary branch may be affected too. It causes:

- vesicular eruptions on the forehead, eyelids and nose of affected side of the face, which crust over
- keratitis
- conjunctivitis.

Complications

- Uveitis.
- Cataract.
- Glaucoma.
- Ophthalmoplegia.
- Persistent pain.
- Ptosis.
- Corneal scarring.
- Anaesthetic cornea.

Tuberculosis

Tuberculosis can cause a uveitis (see p. 123). Rarely miliary tuberculosis causes discrete yellow nodules in the choroid. A retinitis may develop. Phlyctenular conjunctivitis can be caused by tuberculosis.

Sarcoid

Sarcoid can cause a bilateral uveitis (see p. 123) with mutton fat keratic precipitates present on the corneal endothelium. Dry eyes result from sarcoid involvement of the lacrimal gland (see p. 88).

Syphilis

Congenital syphilis can cause interstitial keratitis (see p. 111). It may, rarely, cause a dacryoadenitis.

Acquired syphilis can cause a uveitis and chorioretinitis.

Toxoplasmosis

This is shown in Colour Plate 8.

The toxoplasma parasite can be transmitted in utero if the mother has been infected by ingesting infected meat. It also spreads in the excreta of cats. It causes choroiditis and chorioretinitis (see p. 126).

Toxocara

The toxocara parasite is transmitted via the faeces of puppies and kittens and can cause a unilateral uveitis and choroiditis (see p. 126), affecting children under the age of ten years. A chronic endophthalmitis can occur, resulting in severe loss of vision. It can be treated with Pyrimethamine and steroids.

Rheumatoid arthritis

Rheumatoid arthritis can cause:

- episcleritis (see p. 119)
- scleritis (see p. 119)
- uveitis (see p. 123)
- dry eyes (see p. 88).

Stills disease

Stills disease or juvenile rheumatoid arthritis can cause uveitis (see p. 123).

Ankylosing spondylitis

Ankylosing spondylitis is the main known cause of uveitis (see p. 123) and scleritis (see p. 119).

Ulcerative colitis and Crohn's disease

Ulcerative colitis and Crohn's disease can cause uveitis, scleritis and episcleritis (see pp. 123, 119, and 119 respectively).

Chapter 17
Ophthalmic Drugs

This chapter gives brief details of drugs commonly used in ophthalmic practice.

Mydriatics

Mydriatic drugs are used to dilate the pupil for the following purposes:

- Examination of the retina.
- Maintain dilation of the pupil in uveitis, with corneal ulcers, severe corneal abrasions and after surgery.
- Break down posterior synaechiae which may be present in uveitis.
- Allow a cataract to be extracted.
- Enable retinal surgery to take place.
- Improve vision when a nuclear cataract is present.
- Refraction in children.

There are two groups of mydriatics:

(1) Parasympatholytics, which cause pupillary dilation – mydriasis and cycloplegia – paralysis of the ciliary muscle.
(2) Sympathomimetics, which cause only mydriasis.

Parasympatholytics

G. Atropine sulphate 0.5% or 1%; Oc Atropine sulphate 1%

Derived from the belladonna plant.
Onset: 30 minutes.
Duration: 7–14 days.
Dosage: Usually once or twice a day – may be up to four times.
Side effects can be local or as a result of systemic absorption:

- may cause an allergic reaction
- toxic effects especially in the elderly, including; tachycardia, confusion, drowsiness, hallucinations, thirst.

Disadvantages:

- ○ not readily reversed by miotics
- ○ prolonged duration
- ○ may provoke acute glaucoma in eyes with narrow angles.

G. Homatropine hydrobromide 1% or 2%

A man-made derivative of atropine.
Onset: 30 minutes.
Duration: 24–48 hours.
Dosage: two, three or four times a day.
Advantages:

- can be reversed by pilocarpine
- shorter duration than atropine.

Side effects are similar to those for atropine.

G. Cyclopentolate hydrochloride 0.5% or 1% (Mydrilate)

Onset: 30 minutes.
Duration: 24 hours.
Dosage: two, three or four times a day.
Uses: often used in refraction of children. Pre- and post-operatively.
Side effects are similar to those for atropine.

G. Tropicamide 0.5% or 1% (Mydriacyl)

Onset: 20 minutes.
Duration: six hours.
Dosage: usually only once before examination because of its short-lived effect.
Advantage: short duration makes it suitable for ophthalmoscopy in out-patient or casualty patients.
Side effects are similar to those for atropine.

Sympathomimetics

G. Phenylephrine 2.5%

Onset: 20 minutes.
Duration: three hours.
Dosage: two, three or four times daily, or up to four-hourly to break down posterior synaechiae.
Use: effective in combination with parasympatholytics, especially in the breaking down of posterior synaechiae.
Disadvantages:

- it does not cause cycloplegia
- it can cause corneal epithelial damage
- may cause cardiovascular reactions that may be severe.

Some ophthalmologists may still prescribe G. phenylephrine 10%, but because of side effects it is rarely used.

Notes on mydriatics

- Mydriatics must be used with care in patients who have shallow anterior chambers as dilating the pupils may provoke an attack of closed-angle glaucoma.
- All mydriatics drops sting on instillation to some degree. Phenylephrine usually causes the most discomfort.

Miotics

Miotic drugs constrict the pupil and the ciliary muscle, which opens up the drainage channel for aqueous flow. Therefore their main use is in the treatment of glaucoma.

G. Pilocarpine 0.5%, 1%, 3%, 4% (may be up to 10% in other parts of the world)

A natural compound from the pilocarpes tree found in South America. It is a parasympathomimetic.
Onset: 30 minutes.
Duration: 10–12 hours.
Dosage: two, three or four times a day, or intensively for acute glaucoma.
Disadvantages:

- can cause headaches
- the eye is fixed at accommodation
- the pupil remains permanently miosed, increasing the risk of accidents especially at night as light adaptation is restricted
- care must be taken when used intensively as overdose can cause vomiting
- may cause an allergic reaction
- can sting on instillation.

Acetylcholine chloride 1% (Miochol)

A freshly prepared solution of acetylcholine is injected into the anterior chamber after a cataract extraction to constrict the pupil rapidly to prevent vitreous loss, or to retain a posterior chamber or iris clip intra-ocular lens in position.

Other drugs used in the treatment of glaucoma

Carbonic anhydrase inhibitors

Carbonic anhydrase is an enzyme necessary for the production of aqueous. These drugs therefore cause a reduction in the amount of aqueous produced.

Acetazolamide (Diamox)

Dosage:

- 500 mg intravenously stat in acute glaucoma
- 500 mg orally stat
- 250 mg orally as maintenance four times a day reducing to three or two doses a day or slow release capsules 250 mg given once or twice a day.

Uses: in acute, chronic and secondary glaucoma.

Side effects: drowsiness, gastro-intestinal upset, nausea and potassium loss resulting in tingling of extremities. Potassium supplements such as potassium chloride are sometimes given. It is a weak diuretic.

G. Dorzolamide 2% (Trusopt)

Dosage: three times a day, or twice a day if given with a beta-blocker.
Use: in chronic and secondary glaucoma as an adjuvant therapy to beta-blockers or as a single therapy to non-responders or in those who are unable to tolerate beta-blockers.
Side effects: conjunctivitis, eyelid irritation.

G. Dorzolomide 2% and Timolol 0.5% (Cosopt)

Dosage: twice per day. Timolol is a beta-blocker.
Use: to reduce intra-ocular pressure in open-angle glaucoma.

Beta-blockers

G. Timolol maleate 0.25% or 0.5% (Timoptol)

G. Betaxolol hydrochloride 0.5% (Betoptic)

G. Carteolol hydrochloride 1% or 2% (Teoptic)

G. Levobunolol hydrochloride 0.5% (Betagan)

Actions: reduce the production of aqueous and after several weeks use increase the outflow of aqueous.
Dosage: 12 hourly, strictly (betagan may be used daily).
Advantages: do not cause miosis or accommodation spasm.

Disadvantages: cannot be used in patients with a history of asthma or congestive cardiac failure.

Timolol and levobunolol are available in single dose presentations.

Prostaglandin analogues

Actions: prostaglandin analogues reduce the intra-ocular pressure by increasing the uveoscleral outflow. They are used to treat open angle glaucoma and ocular hypertension.
Disadvantages: the patient needs to be warned that this drug may change the colour of their iris. Caution should be taken if the patient has asthma.
Side effects include: brown pigment on the iris; irritation; lengthening of the eyelashes; peri-orbital oedema; cystoid macular oedema; iritis; uveitis.

G. Latanaprost (Xalatan) 50 μg per ml

Use: once per day, ideally in the evening.

G. Travaprost (Travatan) 40 μg per ml

Use: once per day, ideally in the evening.

G. Bimatoprost (Lumigan) 300 μg per ml

Use: once per day, ideally in the evening.

Other drugs

Mannitol 20%

Use: given intravenously in acute glaucoma when acetazolamide has failed to reduce the intra-ocular pressure. It can be given pre-operatively. Usually 1.5–2 g/kg body weight is given over one hour.

Glycerol

Action: an osmotic.
Use: oral dose given in acute glaucoma when acetazolamide has failed to reduce the intra-ocular pressure.
Dosage: 1.5 g/kg body weight in fruit juice to disguise the taste. It must be drunk within 20 minutes to affect the intra-ocular pressure. Topical glycerol 50% can be used to clear corneal oedema temporarily for ophthalmoscopy to take place.

G. Apraclonidine hydrochloride 0.5% and 1% (Iopidine)

Action: reduces production of aqueous.
Use: adjunctive therapy in chronic glaucoma.

Dosage: three times a day.
Side effects: it is contraindicated in patients with severe or unstable cardio-vascular disease, those receiving monoamine oxidase inhibitors, sympath-omimetic drugs and tricyclic antidepressants. Localised allergy.

Antibiotics

G. Chloramphenicol 0.5%, Oc. 1%

Action: bacteriostatic, broad spectrum.
Uses: in ocular infections. It can penetrate the corneal epithelium. Prophy-lactic use.
Dosage: two-hourly or two, three, or four times a day.
Advantage: resistance is slow to develop.

Gentamicin 0.3% (Genticin) (drops and ointment) 1.5% fortified

Action: bactericidal, broad spectrum.
Uses: ocular infections resistant to chloramphenicol. For *Pseudomonas aerugi-nosa* infections
Dosage: two-hourly or two, three or four times a day. Subconjunctival injec-tion: 10 to 20 mg.

Neomycin sulphate 0.5% (drops and ointment)

Action: bactericidal, broad spectrum.
Uses: in conjunctivitis, blepharitis, superficial infections.
Dosage: two-hourly or two or four times a day.
Disadvantages:

• it does not penetrate corneal tissue
• it may cause an allergic reaction.

Framycetin sulphate 0.5% drops or ointment (Soframycin)

Action, uses and dosage similar to neomycin and therefore can be given in cases allergic to neomycin.

G. Ciprofloxacin 0.3%

Action: broad spectrum antibiotic.
Dosage: intensively for severe infections or two, three or four times a day.
Uses: corneal ulcers, especially caused by pseudomonas.
Side effects: local burning and itching, lid margin crusting.

G. Fucidic acid 1% (Fucithalmic)

Action: broad spectrum antibiotic.
Dosage: usually twice a day.
Uses: superficial infections.
Advantages: a viscous substance that is not absorbed as readily as drops and therefore need not be administered as frequently. Useful in children.

G. Ofloxacin 0.3%

Action: broad spectrum antibiotic.
Dosage: two to four times per day but may be used more frequently if required.

G. Propamidine isethionate 0.1% (Brolene)

Use: in acanthamoeba keratitis.
Dosage: four times a day.
Disadvantage: little value in bacterial conjunctivitis.

Antiviral agents

Oc. Aciclovir (Zovirax) 3%

Dosage: five times a day.
Uses: in herpes simplex virus and herpes zoster ophthalmicus. A cream preparation 5% is available for use on skin lesions.

G. Gancyclovir (Virgan) 0.15%

Dose: five times a day until healed, then three times a day for seven days (21 days total).

Steroids

Steroid drops are used for:

- allergic conditions
- with an antibiotic in bacterial inflammatory conditions, e.g. chronic conjunctivitis
- inflammatory conditions such as uveitis, sympathetic ophthalmia, episcleritis.

G. Prednisolone (Predsol) 0.001%–0.5% (1% Pred. Forte)
Dosage: four times a day.

Methylprednisolone (Depo-Medrone) 20 mg

Dosage: one dose injected onto the orbital floor. Must not be mixed with other drugs in the same syringe.

Betamethasone (Betnesol) G. and Oc. 0.1%

Dosage: two-hourly, two, three or four times a day, ointment at night. 2–4 mg subconjunctivally.

G. Hydrocortisone 1% (ointment 0.5%, 1%, 2.5%)

Dosage: four times a day, ointment at night.

G. Dexamethasone (Maxidex) 0.1%

Dosage: hourly – two-hourly if needed intensively, frequency gradually reducing, or two or four times a day. Must be shaken before instillation.

Neomycin can be combined with a steroid:

Predsol-N (Prednisolone 0.5% and Neomycin 0.5%)

Betnesol-N (Betamethasone 0.1% and Neomycin 0.5%) drops and ointment

Maxitrol (Dexamethasone 0.1%, Neomycin 0.5% and Polymyxin B)

Disadvantages of steroid use

- Lowers the resistance to micro organisms.
- Masks signs of infection.
- Increases the activity of herpes simplex virus.
- May cause herpes simplex viral infection if prescribed for conjunctivitis.
- May cause secondary glaucoma.
- Prolonged use may cause cataract formation.

Local anaesthetics

G. Oxybruprocaine hydrochloride 0.4% (Benoxinate)

Dosage: usually once only is sufficient.
Use: prior to minor ophthalmic procedures.

G. Proxymetacaine 0.5% (Ophthaine)

Dosage: usually once only is sufficient.
Use: minor ophthalmic procedures, often used in children due to reduced stinging on instillation.

G. Tetracaine hydrochloride 0.5% and 1%

Dosage: usually once only is sufficient.
Use: prior to minor ophthalmic procedures.

Diagnostic drops

Fluorescein

Drops: 2%

Uses:

- stains conjunctival and corneal epithelial damage, i.e. corneal ulcers, erosions and conjunctival or corneal abrasions
- assessment of the tear film
- tonometry
- Seidel's test shows fluorescein-stained aqueous leaking from a wound on the cornea/limbus
- contact lens fitting.

Fluorescein is also available in paper strips. Fluorescein should not be dispensed in a multiple container as it is a good medium for *Pseudomonas* bacterial growth.

Intravenous injection: usually 2.5 ml of 25%

Use: for fundal fluorescein angiography, which demonstrates the condition of the retinal blood vessels, the condition of the macula and optic disc and the presence of choroidal tumours.
Disadvantage: discolours the skin and urine.

Indocyanine green (ICG)

Intravenous injection 25 mg in 5 ml of aqueous solvent followed by a bolus dose of normal saline.
Use: highlight retinal and choroidal blood vessels.

Tear replacement

The following are used for dry eyes and must be used as often as is necessary to keep the eyes feeling comfortable. This may be as often as every hour. Once dry eyes have been diagnosed the patient may need to continue to use tear replacement drops for life:

- G. Hypromellose
- G. Tears Naturale

- G. Liquifilm Tears
- G. Viscotears (long-acting gel formulation)
- Simple eye ointment
- Oc. Lacri-Lube
- G. Polyvynyl alcohol (Liquifilm Tears) (Sno Tears)
- G. Povidone (Oculotec).

Miscellaneous

G. Antazoline sulphate 0.5%

Xylometazoline hydrochloride 0.05% (G. Otrivine Antistin)

Use: in allergic conjunctivitis, especially caused by hay fever, for short-term use only.
Dosage: two or three times a day.

G. Sodium cromoglycate (Opticrom) 2%

Use: in allergic conjunctivitis, especially vernal catarrh.
Dosage: four times a day.

G. Lodoxamide (Alomide) 0.1%

Use: in allergic conjunctivitis, as an alternative to Opticrom.
Dosage: four times daily.

G. Olopatadine (Opatanol)

Use: seasonal allergic conjunctivitis.
Dose: twice daily.

Verteporfin (Visudyne)

Use: to treat subfoveal choroidal neovascularisation in wet, age related macular degeneration.
Dose: intravenous infusion based on body mass index. Each eye will require more than one treatment.
Disadvantages: photosensitivity for up to 48 hours. Sunlight, halogen lights and sun beds should be avoided.
Side effects include: blurred vision, flashing lights, field defects, nausea, vomiting, fever, back pain, hypertension.

Sodium hyaluronate (Healonid)

A visco-elastic polymer normally present in aqueous.
Use: during surgical procedures to protect internal structures and maintain depth of anterior chamber.

Side effects: occasional hypersensitivity, transient rise in intra-ocular pressure.

Botulinum toxin (clostridium botulinum type A; Dysport, Botox)

Action: paralysis of muscles.
Use: to treat blepharospasm and strabismus and to induce ptosis to protect the cornea.
Dosage: varies depending on use and which product is used.
Side effects: as it is a biological product, anaphylaxis may occur.

G. Diclofenac sodium 0.1% (Volterol Ophtha)

Use: inhibits intra-operative miosis, reduces post-cataract surgery inflammation.
Dosage:

   pre-operative: $^1/_2$ hourly four times
   post-operative: four times a day.

Advantage: preservative-free preparation.

General note

Many ophthalmic drugs are prepared in single-dose containers that contain no preservative. Therefore they are useful for those patients who may be allergic to the preservative used in ophthalmic preparations.

Appendix 1: Correction of Refractive Errors

Light travels in rays that are reflected from objects into the eyes. Light rays travel in straight lines from a distance of 6 metres or more. At a shorter distance they diverge as they enter the eye. When light rays meet a transparent object at an angle they bend. This is called 'refraction'. Light rays entering the eye meet the curved cornea and bend inwards or converge. They continue to converge as they pass through each of the refractive media of the eye, the cornea, the aqueous, the lens and the vitreous, so that they are brought to a focal point on the retina (American Academy of Ophthalmology 2003/2004).

The 'refractive power' of the eye is the degree to which the eye is able to refract the light rays. This power is expressed in dioptres. One dioptre brings rays of light to a focus over one metre. Ten dioptres bring rays of light to a focus over one-tenth of a metre or 10 cm. The refractive power of the eye is 60 dioptres. (that of the lens is 20 dioptres and of the cornea 40 dioptres).

Long sight or hypermetropia

A long-sighted person has a short eyeball. The light rays therefore come to a focus behind the retina causing blurred vision. A long-sighted person consequently has to accommodate for their distant vision to be clear. No further accommodation is possible for near vision, so this is blurred. If a convex lens is placed in front of the eye, the light rays will converge more sharply and come to a focus on the retina. A convex lens is a spherical lens because its shape is equal in all meridians. It is known as a 'plus' lens.

Short sight or myopia

A short-sighted person has a long eyeball. The light rays therefore come to a focus in front of the retina. The vision is usually more blurred for distant vision than near vision as the lens can accommodate for near vision. If a concave lens is placed in front of the eye, the light rays will diverge before converging through the cornea and lens and will come to a focus at the retina. A concave lens is also spherical and is known as a 'minus' lens.

Iris claw lenses have been placed in phacic eyes above −6.00 dioptres myopia with successful results (Menezo et al., 1995).

Presbyopia

From the age of about 45 years, the lens in the eye no longer has the ability to accommodate for near vision. The light rays therefore fall behind the retina before coming to a focus. This is known as presbyopia. Convex or plus lenses are needed to bring the image into focus on the retina. An increasingly powerful lens is required until the age of 70 years when no further deterioration in focusing occurs.

Astigmatism

The astigmatic cornea has an uneven curvature so that there is no point of focus of the light rays on the retina. A cylindrical lens placed in front of the eye with its axis corresponding to the abnormal plane on the cornea will focus the light rays. The cylindrical lens can either be concave or convex.

Most spectacles combine both spherical (plus or minus) lenses with cylindrical lenses to provide a compound lens to correct myopia/hypermetropia and astigmatism. Full information on optics is beyond the scope of this book.

Correction techniques

The main principle of correcting refractive errors is to modify the refractive power. Correction of refractive errors can be made in a variety ways listed below.

Spectacles

Spectacles are still the most widely used and are universally the safest devices. However for various reasons, some people find spectacles unacceptable and not necessarily the answer to their vision problems. For example, wearing spectacles in some working environments can be hazardous; others find glasses impractical for some sports like rugby or football; and for others they are cosmetically unacceptable.

Contact lenses

Contact lenses are more popular as they provide convenience, are reasonably safe but not risk free. Usually contact lenses can either be gas permeable or soft lenses. Soft lenses can be daily or monthly disposable or extended wear. Users of contact lenses can encounter problems such as eye infections, abrasions, chemical injury (as a result of inadvertently using contact lens cleaner instead of the wetting solution), corneal ulcers and problems of over wearing their lenses. Contact lenses wearers must visit their opticians for regular eye check if problems are to be avoided. Cleaning guidelines must be strictly adhered to. However, some people cannot tolerate contact lenses either because of dry eyes, allergy to the solution or to the lenses themselves. Certain environments such as very dusty or smoky surroundings make wearing of contact lenses intolerable.

Refractive surgery

In recent years there has been an increased interest in refractive surgery. Initially this was performed for myopia, but recent advances have enabled patients with hypermetropia and astigmatism also to be treated. It is still at an early stage of development and the long-term results are unknown. There is a degree of controversy and caution about the process (Gartry, 1995).

Radial keratotomy

This operation consists of radial incisions involving 90% of the corneal thickness (Vaughan et al., 1999) near towards the limbus. Radial keratotomy is more successful in individuals who are within the myopic range of –2 to –4. Side effects such as fluctuations of vision and glare have been reported. Corneal infections as a result of delayed healing of the corneal incisions is another complication.

Laser photorefractive keratectomy (PRK)

Laser photorefractive keratectomy has largely replaced redial keratotomy. In PRK, the corena is subjected to light energy from the excimer laser to excise tissue from the cornea. A computer estimates the depth and position of the corneal tissue to be removed which will vary depending on the refractive error being treated. The energy from the laser beam is subjected to the central cornea with resultant flattening of the cornea. The Bowman's memebrane is removed during PRK which can sometimes produce a corneal haze.

Shortcomings of the procedure are:

- Visual results are better predicted in patients whose refractive error is less than –6 dioptres than higher myopes (–6 to –10). However, higher myopes can obtain a reduction in their myopia (Carson & Taylor, 1995).
- Severe pain while the epithelium regenerates.
- Complications include: corneal haze which is significantly more in myopes greater than –10 (Carson & Taylor, 1995), regression, loss of best corrected visual acuity, night halo effects, wound infection, delayed healing and perforation.

Laser in-situ keratomileusis (LASIK)

This is a surgical procedure to correct myopia, hypermetropia and astigmatism which utilises a microkeratome to create a corneal 'flap' of about one-third of the total corneal thickness. The thickness of the flap is dependent on the degree of myopia to be corrected and the individual's corneal thickness. The flap is reflected towards the hinge. The excimer laser is focused and centered on the exposed middle layer of the cornea. When laser treatment is completed, the flap is swept back into position.

The patient is usually seen the next day following surgery to measure the visual acuity, to inspect flap position and to ensure that no signs of infection or inflammation are present. A broad spectrum antibiotic such as Ofloxacin is prescribed. However the consensus on the use of steroids does not exist.

Patient's needs

- The patient must have detailed explanations given of the procedure itself and any complications.
- Topography investigations: the curvature of the cornea is measured in detail resulting in a coloured map of the cornea. Areas that are too flat are coloured blue and those too steep red. The ideal curvature is green.
- Pre- and post-operative care.
- Follow-up information.

Nursing action

- Assist/perform topography.
- Ensure the patient has a full understanding of the procedure and that he does not have unrealistic expectations.
- Give pre-operative care. Local anaesthetic drops will be instilled.
- Assist in the laser surgery.
- Give post-operative care:
  - a bandage contact lens will be in place (see p. 245)
  - ensure the patient has adequate analgesia
  - ensure the patient has follow-up information including understanding that if treated for myopia, he will initially be hypermetropic

Paralytic squint

When a paralytic squint occurs, the image to each eye is not focusing on the same area of each retina. If a prism is placed in front of the squinting eye, the light rays bend towards the base of the triangular-shaped prismatic lens and will cause the image to focus in the area of the retina of that eye corresponding to the area of retina in the other eye. This results in a single image being seen or binocular single vision.

Appendix 2: Contact Lenses

Uses of contact lenses

- Refractive errors: people may wear contact lenses for cosmetic reasons instead of glasses. High myopes benefit from wearing contact lenses because they would need to wear thick-lensed glasses which cause visual distortion. Contact lenses afford much improved vision involving the whole visual field.
- Aphakia (see p. 156).
- Corneal abnormalities such as keratoconus (see p. 112).
- Protection: a bandage lens can protect the eye from perforating or becoming too dry. Painted contact lenses are worn by albinos or people with aniridia to prevent too much light entering the eye.
- Some people seek to have myopia corrected by the insertion of an intra-ocular lens surgically so they do not have to wear glasses or contact lenses.

Types of lens

- Hard or rigid lens.
- Gas-permeable lens.
- Soft lens.
- Extended-wear lens.
- Bandage lens.
- Disposable – monthly/weekly/daily.
- Toric and bi-toric for astigmatism.
- Bifocal.

Hard and gas-permeable lenses

Hard and gas-permeable lenses must be removed before sleep or if the eye is irritable. If they are kept in under these circumstances, corneal damage is likely to occur. Artificial teardrops may be required to prevent the cornea drying out. Gas-permeable lenses should cause less corneal dryness.

Soft lenses

Soft lenses are slightly larger than hard lenses. They tend to be used if the wearer finds hard lenses intolerable. They should also be removed at night and if the eye is irritable. More scrupulous care is required for soft lenses as they are more likely to cause corneal damage; because they are made of a softer material than hard lenses, a scratch on the cornea or a small foreign body underneath the lens is not so likely to be felt until damage has been done.

Fluorescein drops should never be put into an eye with a soft contact lens in, as the dye will be taken up by the lens and is extremely difficult, if not impossible, to remove. Only eye drops without preservative should be used with soft contact lenses, as the preservative can be absorbed by the lens, which may provoke an allergic reaction. Soft lenses should be stored in normal saline if no soaking solution is available; water, whether sterile or not, will cause them to dry out.

Extended-wear lenses and bandage lenses

Extended-wear lenses and bandage lenses are essentially similar to soft lenses but are larger in size. They can be worn for up to three months without being removed, so are therefore useful for the young and the elderly. The optician removes the lens and replaces it with a new one. Artificial teardrops will be required to prevent the cornea drying out.

Bandage lenses do not have a prescription incorporated.

Disposable monthly/weekly/daily lenses

Disposable lenses are becoming more popular. Initially the lenses were designed to be worn day and night for six days and then discarded. The eyes were rested on the seventh day. Some contact lens wearers now use disposable lenses but as daily wear, removing them at night to reduce the complications (see p. 246).

Care of contact lenses

Contact lenses require great care to prevent corneal damage and eye infection. There are several different brands of products on the market for use with contact lenses. Two important steps in the care of the lenses are handwashing before and after handling the lenses and cleaning the contact lens case. There are different solutions for hard and soft lenses.

Care of lenses involves:

- Cleansing with a cleansing solution rubbed on the lens with the finger and washed off with water. It has been suggested that using solutions containing hydrogen peroxide are better in that they destroy acanthamoeba (see p. 246).

- Wetting – wetting solution is dropped onto the corneal surface of the lens before it is inserted into the eye.
- Soaking the lens – when the lens is not in the eye, i.e. overnight, it is placed in a special container filled with soaking solution. This fluid should be changed each time the container is used. Once a week the container should be washed out with warm water and rinsed with the soaking solution.
- There are now 'all in one' solutions available that reduce the number of processes involved in the care process. By doing so it is hoped that the wearer will better comply with a simple regimen.

Lenses should be cleaned well and checked by an optician before being re-inserted following corneal damage.

Insertion/removal of contact lenses

See p. 44 for details of how to insert and remove contact lenses.

Complications of contact lens wear

- Intolerance: some people find wearing contact lenses intolerable. Hard lenses are usually prescribed initially as they cause less problems. If these are difficult to wear, gas-permeable or soft contact lenses are prescribed. Some people have to abandon contact lens wearing and resort to spectacles.
- Corneal abrasion.
- Dry eyes: the lens prevents the tear film from adequately covering the cornea. Artificial teardrops can be prescribed for people who do experience dry eyes.
- Giant papillary conjunctivitis or contact lens associated papillary conjunctivitis. This is more common in wearers of soft contact lenses. It may not manifest itself for months or years after starting to wear lenses. Symptoms include:
  o   itching
  o   mucus discharge
  o   increasing intolerance to lens wear.

Signs: large conjunctival papillae (Kanski, 2003).

- Hypoxia: the cornea is deprived of oxygen from the tear film by the presence of the contact lens. The cornea becomes oedematous and new vessels may develop in the limbal area. This usually occurs after years of contact lens wear.
- Sensitivity: this may develop in response to the preservative in the cleaning and soaking solutions.

- Keratitis: people wearing extended-wear soft contact lenses are 21 times more likely to get microbial keratitis than gas-permeable lens wearers and daily soft contact lens wearers are four times more likely to suffer from keratitis at some point (Cochrane, 1993). Acanthamoeba is the most dangerous organism requiring intensive antibiotic application (Kanski, 2003). This may be Chlorhexidine and Polyhexamethylenebinguanide. The contact lens should not be reinserted into the eye until the infection has cleared and the lens itself has been cleaned.

It is advisable for all contact lens wearers to have a spare pair of spectacles to wear in case they are unable to use their contact lenses for a while.

Nurse's role

Although nurses do not prescribe or fit contact lenses, they are in an ideal position to educate people on the care of contact lenses whether the person has a problem or in a more informal advisory capacity.

Nurses must stress the importance of the following:

- Complying with scrupulous and effective care regimes of their contact lenses (Wakelin, 1995; American Academy of Ophthalmologists, 2003). However, wearers of extended-wear soft contact lenses have an increased risk of keratitis despite complying with hygiene instructions (Stapleton, 1992).
- The need to discard any remaining solution after 28 days of use.
- Saliva and tap water must not be used as wetting or cleaning solutions.
- Other people's contact lens cases, which may not be clean, must not be 'borrowed' for their lenses.
- Allowing time for the cornea to 'breathe' by removing the lenses for a period of time each day.
- Removal of lenses, except extended-wear lenses, at night.
- Washing of hands prior to handling lenses and avoiding creamy soft soaps and ensuring all traces of hand cream are removed from finger tips.
- Avoiding swimming/jacuzzis whilst wearing contact lenses.
- Removing the lenses if the eye becomes sore and seeking medical advice.
- Remove contact lenses before going to sleep.

Glossary

Abduction Turning the eye outwards.

Acanthamoeba A genus of free-living amoeba.

Accommodation The ability of the lens to change shape to allow near objects to be focused on the retina.

Acne rosacea Disease of the skin characterised by bullous nose and erythema of the cheeks, forehead and nose.

Adduction Turning the eye inwards.

Afferent pupil defect A defect of the pupillary reflex in which shining a light in the affected eye will result in a dilatation of the pupil. This condition is due to an optic nerve lesion.

Amblyopia Reduced vision usually due to interference with the eye's development.

Angles Alpha, Kappa and Gamma Different angles in the eye measured between the optic axis and the visual axis.

Aniridia Absence of the iris.

Aphakia Absence of the lens.

Applanation tonometry Measurement of the intra-ocular pressure by flattening the cornea.

Arcus senilis Degenerative change in the cornea resulting in a white ring around the corneal circumference.

Argon laser Laser that uses photocoagulation.

Astigmatism Uneven curvature of the cornea.

Binocular vision Co-ordinated use of both eyes resulting in a single vision.

Biometry Measurement of the axial length of the eye (A-scan).

Blepharitis Inflammation of the lid margin.

Blepharospasm Painful involuntary spasm of the eyelids.

Blind spot Optic disc where there are no nerve endings, only nerve fibres.

Bullous keratopathy Oedema of the cornea causing 'blister' formation in the epithelium.

Buphthalmos Congenital glaucoma.

Burkitt's lymphoma A malignant tumour of the lympathetic system affecting mainly children.

Canthus Outer and inner areas where the upper and lower lids meet.

Capsulotomy Opening of the capsule of the lens.

Cartella shield Plastic shield to protect the eye.

Caruncle Small fleshy area in inner corner of the eye.

Cataract   Opacity of the lens.

Central field/vision   Area of vision when looking straight ahead.

Chalazion   Meibomian gland cyst. Internal hordeolum.

Chemosis   Oedema of the conjunctiva.

Chlamydia   Chronic conjunctivitis caused by serotypes D–K of *Chlamydia trachomatis*.

Commotio retinae   Oedema of the retina following trauma.

Concave lens   A lens which diverges light rays, used to correct myopia: a 'minus' lens.

Concretion   Lipid deposit in the conjunctiva.

Convex lens   A lens which converges light rays, used to correct hypermetropia: a 'plus' lens.

Cool laser   Procedure similar to phacoemulsification but uses 'cool laser' shock waves to fragment the lens.

Cover test   A test for determining the presence of phoria or trophia.

Cycloplegia   Paralysis of the ciliary muscles.

Cylindrical lens   A lens of cylindrical shape, which refracts light rays in various directions in different meridians, used to correct astigmatism.

Dacryoadenitis   Inflammation of the lacrimal gland.

Dacryocystitis   Inflammation of the lacrimal sac.

Dacryocystorhinostomy   An operation to make a passage from the lacrimal sac into the nose to overcome an obstruction.

Dendritic ulcer   A branching ulcer of the cornea caused by the herpes simplex virus.

Descemetocele   Protrusion of Descemet's membrane through the stroma and epithelium of the cornea.

Dioptre   Unit of measurement of strength of the refractive power of the eye, or lenses, expressed as a fraction of a metre.

Diplopia   Double vision.

Disciform keratitis   Inflammation of the cornea as a complication of herpes simplex virus.

Distichiasis   Double row of eyelashes.

Drusen   Small yellow nodule in Bruch's membrane, or optic nerve.

Ectropion   Turning out of the eyelid.

Electroretinogram   A recording of electrical activity of the retina.

Emmetropia   Absence of refractive error.

Endophthalmitis   Inflammation/infection of inner structures of the eye.

Enophthalmos   Displacement of the eyeball downwards.

Entropion   Turning inwards of the lid margin.

Enucleation   Removal of the eyeball and length of optic nerve.

Epicanthus   Broad fold of skin in inner canthus.

Epilation   Removal of an eyelash.

Epiphora   Watering eye.

Episcleritis   Inflammation of the episcleral vessels.

Evisceration   Removal of the contents of the eyeball, leaving the sclera intact.

Excimer laser   Laser used for corneal surgery, e.g. for correcting refractive errors or removing corneal scars.

Exenteration   Removal of the contents of the orbit, including the eyeball and lids.

Exophthalmometer   Instrument for measuring the degree of protrusion of an eye.

Exophthalmos   Protrusion of one or both eyes – usually refers to that caused by thyroid eye disease.

Extracapsular lens extraction   Removal of the anterior lens capsule, the cortex and nucleus but leaving the posterior lens capsule intact.

Field of vision   The entire area that can be seen without moving the eye.

Fields of gaze   The different areas that can be seen when moving the eye in all directions.

Fixation   The eyes are fixed on an object centrally at a chosen distance.

Floaters   Small, dark particles in the vitreous.

Follicles   Dome shaped elevations on the palpebral conjunctiva containing lymphocytes. Follicles are avascular.

Fresnel prism   Thin transparent plastic disc which is attached to a pair of glasses to eliminate diplopia.

Fuch's dystrophy   Disorder of the descemet membrance of the cornea with wart like deposits and thickening. Defect in the endotheliun is also noted.

Fundus   Posterior aspect of the retina including the optic disc and the macula.

Fusion   Co-ordinating the images seen by both eyes into a single image.

Glaucoma   A group of conditions characterised by an increased intra-ocular pressure sufficient to damage vision.

Gonioscope   A contact lens mirror used to view the anterior chamber angle.

Guttae   (G.) Eyedrops.

Hemianopia   Half-vision – unilateral or bilateral.

Heterochromia   Different coloured irises in one person.

Hess chart   A chart for measuring and classifying strabismus.

Hordeolum   Internal, see Chalazion; external, see Stye.

Hydroxyapatite implant   Derived material from coral used as an implant in enucleation.

Hypermetropia   Long sight.

Hyphaema   Blood in the anterior chamber.

Hypopyon   Pus in the anterior chamber.

Indocyanine green   Newer dye than fluorescein sodium which gives better information on the choroidal circulation and is particularly helpful in the diagnosis of choroidal neovascular membrances.

Imber-Fick law   States that the intra-ocular pressure (P in mmHg) is equal to the tonometer weight (W) divided by the applanated area of the cornea. This is applicable for applanation tonometry.

Injection   Degree of redness of the conjunctiva.

Interpupillary distance (IPD)   The distance between the two pupils.

Intracapsular lens extraction   Removal of the entire lens including the anterior and posterior capsules.

Interstitial keratitis   Inflammation of the cornea due to syphilis.
Iridectomy   Removal of a piece of the iris.
Iridodialysis   Severance of the iris from the ciliary body.
Iridodonesis   Quivering of iris following intra-capsular cataract extraction.
Iridotomy   A hole in the iris, usually performed by the laser beam.
Iris bombe   Bulging forward of the iris.
Iris prolapse   A section of the iris prolapsing through a wound, either surgical or traumatic.
Iritis   Inflammation of the iris.
Ishihara colour plates   Multicoloured charts for testing colour vision.
Kaposi's sarcoma   Vascular tumour of HIV patients appearing as multiple purple to red nodules on the skin and mucous membrances.
Keratitic precipitates   Plaques of protein adhered to the corneal endothelium in uveitis.
Keratitis   Inflammation of the cornea.
Keratoconus   Conical-shaped deformity of the cornea.
Keratometer   Instrument for measuring the curvature of the cornea.
Lacrimation   Production of tears.
Lagophthalmos   Incomplete closure of the eyelids.
Lamellar graft   Partial thickness corneal graft.
Laser Light   Amplification by stimulated emission of radiation. Energy transmitted as heat.
Laser in situ keratomileusis (LASIK)   A surgical procedure to correct myopia, hypermetropia and astigmatism by creating a corneal flap.
Lensectomy   Removal of the entire lens and capsule including an anterior segment of the vitreous using specialised equipment.
Molluscum contagiosum   Viral infection of the skin occuring on the face or eyelids manifested by a shiny, raised skin nodule.
Microphthalmos   Small eyeball.
Miotic   Drug that constricts the pupil.
Mydriatic   Drug that dilates the pupil.
Myopia   Short sight.
Needling   A procedure used to remove soft lens matter on an infant or child.
Occulentum (Oc.)   Eye ointment.
Operculum   A semi-circular tear in the retina, covered with a flap of retina.
Ophthalmia neonatorum   Severe conjunctivitis of the newborn.
Ophthalmoplegia   Paralysis of the extra-ocular muscles.
Ophthalmoscope   Instrument for examining the retina.
Optic axis   The line through the centre of the optical structures of the eye.
Osteo-odonto-keraprosthesis surgery   A type of surgical technique where patient's own tooth root and aveolar bone are used instead of conventional corneal graft technique.
Pachymetry   A technique to measure the corneal thickness by using a pachometer.
Palpebral   Pertaining to the eyelids.
Papillae   Tiny elevation seen on palpebral conjunctiva with vascular cores.

Pemphigoid An autoimmune disease of the elderly characterised by chronic itchy blistering usually on the limbs.

Pannus Neovascularisation of the cornea.

Panophthalmitis Inflammation of the whole eyeball.

Penetrating graft Full-thickness corneal graft.

Perimeter Instrument for measuring the field of vision.

Peripheral vision/field Area of vision outside central field of vision.

PGD Patient group directions.

Phacoemulsification Removal of cataract by ultrasound, breaking down lens matter prior to it being aspirated.

Phacolytic lens Lens matter leaking out giving rise to uveitis and secondary glaucoma.

Phasing Regular frequent measurements of intra-ocular pressure over a few days.

Phlyctenule Small vesicle of allergic origin on limbal area of conjunctiva and/or cornea.

Photophobia Sensitivity to light.

Photopsia Sensation of flashing lights.

Photorefractive keratectomy (PRK) Correction of refractive errors using excimer laser.

Phthisis bulbi Shrunken eyeball.

Pinguecula A yellowish overgrowth of conjunctiva.

Placido's disc A disc with alternating black and white rings for reflecting onto the cornea to detect any irregularity in its curvature.

Presbyopia Inability to focus for near sight due to hardening of the lens nucleus after the age of 40 years.

Preseptal callulitis Inflammation of preseptal portion of eyelids.

Prism A triangular-shaped lens used to correct diplopia.

Proptosis Protrusion of the eyeball.

Pterygium A triangular proliferation of conjunctival tissue that can invade the cornea.

Ptosis Drooping eyelid.

Radial keratotomy A surgical procedure consisting of radial incisions to the cornea used to correct myopia.

Refraction (1) Bending of light rays; (2) Measurement of and correction of refractive errors of the eye.

Refractive surgery Corneal surgery to correct refractive errors.

Reiter's syndrome A condition characterised by inflammation of the conjunctiva, urethra and polyarthritis. This condition usually affects young males.

Retinal detachment Separation of the epithelial layer of the retina from its neural layers.

Retinitis pigmentosa A hereditary degeneration of the retina.

Retinoblastoma Highly malignant tumour of the retina in infancy.

Retinopathy Non-inflammatory disease of the retina.

Retinopathy of prematurity A vasoproliferative retinopathy occurring in premature infants.

Retinoscope   Instrument for objective assessment of refractive errors.

Retrobulbar   Behind the eyeball.

Retropunctal cautery   Cautery applied behind the punctum to cause fibrosis and inturning of the lower lid.

Rhodopsin   Light-sensitive pigment of the rods in the retina – 'visual purple'.

Rodding of fornices   Passing a glass rod in either fornix.

Rubeosis irides   Neovascularisation of the iris.

Scleritis   Inflammation of the sclera.

Scleromalacia   Degeneration of the sclera.

Scotoma   An area of visual loss in the visual field.

Siedel test   A test to ascertain leakage of aqueous through a section or perforative wound using fluorescein drops.

Sturge-Weber syndrome   Red discolouration of the skin often referred to as 'port wine stain' which is present at birth and which is permanent.

Sjögren's syndrome   Syndrome comprising arthritis, dry eyes, dysphagia and achlorhydria.

Snellen chart   A chart consisting of graded letters, symbols or numbers for testing central vision.

Specular photomicroscopy   Special mounted slit lamp camera which allows the corneal endothelium to be photographed and counted.

Squint Strabismus   Deviation of one eye.

Staphyloma   A protrusion of the cornea or sclera.

Stereopsis   Perception of depth with binocular vision.

Stevens–Johnson syndrome   Acute mucocutaneous vesiculobullous disease.

Strabismus   See Squint.

Stye   Inflammation of one lash follicle. External hordeolum.

Superficial punctate keratitis   Superficial spots of inflammation of the cornea which stain with G. fluorescein.

Symblephron   Adhesion of the bulbar and palpebral conjunctiva.

Sympathetic ophthalmitis   Severe uveitis in one eye following trauma involving the uvea of the other eye.

Synaechiae adhesion of the iris   (a) to the lens – posterior synaechiae; (b) to the cornea – anterior synaechiae.

Tarsorrhaphy   Suturing together of the eyelids.

Tear film   The film of fluid covering the eyeball.

Tenon's capsule   Membrane encircling globe from limbus to optic nerve overlying the sclera.

Tomography   Computerised scan of the optic disc.

Tonometer   Instrument for measuring intra-ocular pressure.

Topography   A contour map of the curvature of the cornea.

Toric contact lens   Contact lens to correct astigmatism.

Trachoma   Potentially blinding infection of the conjunctiva and cornea caused by the TRIC virus.

Trichiasis   Ingrowing or inturning of eyelashes.

Uveitis   Inflammation of the uveal tract.

Visual acuity   Detailed central vision.

Visual axis   The line between a point viewed and the macula.

Visual field   Area of vision.

Vitrectomy   Removal of vitreous.

Xanthelasma   Fatty deposits on the eyelids.

Xerophthalmia   Lack of vitamin A resulting in corneal and conjunctival disease.

Yag laser   Laser that cuts holes in structures.

References and Further Reading

Allen, M., Knight, C., Falk, C. and Strong, V. (1992) Effectiveness of a pre-operative teaching program for cataract patients. *Journal of Advanced Nursing*, **17**, 303–09.

American Academy of Ophthalmology (2003/2004) *Optics, Refraction and Contact Lenses*. AAO, San Francisco.

Anon (1995) Focus – the cornea-plastic unit. *Eye News*, **1**(2), 20–21.

Barker, B. (1985) *Patient Assessment in Psychiatric Nursing*. Croom Helm, London.

Beare, J.D.L. (1990) Eye injuries from assault with chemicals. *British Journal of Ophthalmology*, **74**, 514–18.

Bonner, E., Dowling, S. and Eustace, P. (1994) A survey of blepharitis in pre-operative cataract patients. *European Journal of Implant and Refractive Surgery*, **6**, 87–92.

Brady, K., Scott Atkinson, L., Kilby, L. and Hilary, D. (1995) Cataract surgery and intraocular lens implantation in children. *American Journal of Ophthalmology*, **120**(1), 1–9.

Brahma, A., Shah, S., Hiller, V., Mcleod, D., Sabala, T., Brown, A. and Marsden, J. (1996) Topical analgesia for superficial corneal injuries. *Journal of Accident & Emergency Medicine*, **1**(3), 186–88.

British Medical Association & Royal Pharmaceutical Society of Great Britain (2004) *British National Formulary*. BMA, London.

British Thoracic Society (2004) http://www.brit-thoracic.org.uk/public

Broadway, D., Grierson, I., O'Brien, C. and Hutchings, R. (1994) Adverse effects of topical antiglaucoma medication. *Archives of Ophthalmology*, **112**, 1437–45.

Bruce, I., McKennel, A. and Walker, E. (1991) *Blind and Partially Sighted Adults in Britain*. The Royal National Institute for the Blind Survey, HMSO, London.

Budenz, D.L., Barton, K. and Tseng, S.C. (2000) Amniotic membrane transplantation for repair of leaking glaucoma for filtering blebs. *American Journal of Ophthalmology*, **130**, 580–88.

Carson, C. and Taylor, H. (1995) Excimer laser treatment for high and extreme myopia. *Archives of Ophthalmology*, **113**, 431–36.

Cochrane, C. (1993) Contact lenses and bacterial injections. *Nursing Standard*, **7**(20), 32–34.

Collin, R. and Rose, G. (2001) *Fundamentals of Clinical Ophthalmology – Plastic and Orbital Surgery*. BMJ Books, London.

Conway, J. (1994) Reflection – the art and science of nursing and the theory practice gap. *British Journal of Nursing*, **3**(3), 114–18.

Corbett, M.C., Rosen, E.S. and O'Bratt, D.P.S. (1999) *Corneal Topography: Principles and applications*. BMJ Books, London.

Damato, B. (1995) Ten FAQs on the management of uveal melanomas. *Eye News*, **1**(5), 5–7.

Davies, P., Bailey, P.J., Goldeberg, M. and Ford Hutchinson, A.W. (1984) The role of arachidonic acid oxygenation products in pain and inflammation. *Annual Review of Immunology* **2**, 335–57.

De Rott, A. (1940) Plastic repair of conjunctival defects with fetal membranes. *Archives of Ophthalmology*, **23**, 522–25.

Dhilton, B. and Millar, G. (1994) *The Child's Eye: Diagnosis of Ophthalmic Disorders in Children*. Oxford Medical Publications, New York.

DoH (2000) *NHS Plan*. Department of Health, HMSO, London.

DoH (2003) *Essence of Care*. Department of Health, HMSO, London.

Duker, J. and Tolentino, F. (1991) Retinopathy of prematurity and pediatric retina and vitreous disorders. *Current Opinion in Ophthalmology*, **2**, 690–95.

Dutton, J.J. (1991) Coralline hydroxyapatite ocular implant. *Ophthalmology*, **98**(3), 370–77.

Elder, M.J. (1994) Combined trabeculotomy – trabeculectomy compared with primary trabeculectomy for congenital glaucoma. *British Journal of Ophthalmology*, **78**(10), 745–48.

Engstrom, R. and Holland, G. (1995) Local therapy for cytomegalovirus retinopathy. *American Journal of Ophthalmology*, **120**(3), 376–85.

Field, D., Martin, D. and Witchell, L. (1999) Ophthalmic chloramphenicol: friend or foe. *International Journal of Ophthalmic Nursing*, **2**(4), 4–7.

Forrester, J.V., Dick, A.D., McMenamin, P.G. and Lee, W.R. (2002) *The Eye. Basic Sciences in Practice, 2nd edition*. W. B. Saunders, Edinburgh.

Gartry, D.S. (1995) Treating myopia with the excimer laser. The present position. *British Medical Journal*, **310**, 979–85.

Hersch, P., Rice, B. and Baer, J. (1990) Topical non-steroidals agents and corneal wound healing. *Archives of Ophthalmology*, **108**, 577–83.

Hope-Ross, M., Yannuzzi, L.A., Gragoudas, E.S. et al. (1994) Adverse reactions due to indocyanine green. *Ophthalmology*, **101**(3), 529–33.

Jabs, D., Grell, R., Fox, R. and Bartlett, J. (1989) Ocular manifestations of acquired immunodeficiency syndrome. *Ophthalmology*, **96**(7), 1092–99.

Jayamanne, D., Fitt, A., Dayan, M., Andrews, R., Mitchell, K. and Griffiths, P. (1997) The effectiveness of topical diclofenac in relieving discomfort following traumatic corneal abrasions. *Eye*, **11**, 79–83.

Jones, C.A. Socket surgery. In: (2001) *Plastic and Orbital Surgery* (R. Collin and G. Rose). BMJ Books, London.

Jones, N.P. (1998) *Uveitis – an illustrated manual*. Butterworth Heinemann, Oxford.

Jose, R., Faria de Abreu, J.R., Silva, R. and Cunha-Vaz, J.G. (1994) The blood–retinal barrier in diabetes during pregnancy. *Archives of Ophthalmology*, **112**, 1334–38.

Kanski, J. (2003) *Clinical Ophthalmology*, 5th edition. Butterworth Heinemann, Oxford.

Kanski, J.J., McAllister, J.A. and Salmon, J.F. (1996) *Glaucoma. A Colour Manual of Diagnosis and Treatment*, 2nd edition. Butterworth Heinemann, Oxford.

Kirkpatrick, J., Hoh, H. and Cook, S. (1993) No eye pad for corneal abrasions. *Eye*, **7**(5), 468–71.

Kuppens, E., Van Best, J. and Sterk, C. (1995) Is glaucoma associated with an increased risk of contact? *British Journal of Ophthalmology*, **79**(7), 649–52.

Kyngas, H., Duffy, M.E. and Kroll, T. (2000) Conceptual analysis of compliance. *Journal of Clinical Nursing*, **9**, 5–12.

Laske, M., Connel, A. and Schacchat, A. et al. (1994) The Barbados eye study, prevalence of open-angle glaucoma. *Archives of Ophthalmology*, **112**, 821–29.

Latham, B., Higgins, L. and Ambrose, P. (1992) Cataract patient's post-operative eye care: development and evaluation of a teaching program. *Australian Journal of Advanced Nursing*, **10**(1), 4–8.

Lee, S.H. and Tseng, S.C.G. (1997) Amniotic membrane transplantation for severe neurotropic ulcers. *British Journal of Ophthalmology*, **123**, 302–03.

Leske, C.M., Heijl, A., Hussein, M., Benbtsson, B., Hyman, L. and Komaroff, E. (2003) Factors for Glaucoma progression and the effect of Treatment. *Archives of Ophthalmology*, **121**, 48–56.

Lund-Johansen, P. (1990) The dye dilution method for measurement of cardiac output. *European Heart Journal*, **11**(suppl I), 6–12.

Manchester Royal Eye Hospital (2004) *Protocol for the management of POAG*. MREH, Manchester.

Martin, O., Parks, D. and Mellows, S. et al. (1994) Treatment of cytomegalovirus retinitis with sustained-release ganciclovir implant. *Archives of Ophthalmology*, **112**, 1531–39.

McBride, S. (2000) *Patients talking*. RNIB, London.

McBride, S. (2002) *Patients talking 2*. RNIB, London.

McDonald, S. (1998) Unpublished paper on the use of ketorolac tromethamine in the treatment of corneal pain. Westbourne Eye Hospital, Bournemouth.

McGarey, B.E., Napalkav, J.A., Pippen, P.A. and Reaves, T.A. (1993) Corneal wound healing strength with topical anti-inflammatory drugs (ARVO abstracts). *Invest Ophthalmol Vis Sci* **1321**.

McNicholl, C. (1995) Phacoemulsification. *British Journal of Nursing*, **5**(2), 22–24.

Menezo, J., Cisneros, A. and Hueso, J. et al. (1995) Long-term results of surgical treatment of high myopia with Worst-Fechner intraocular lenses. *Journal of Cataract and Refractive Surgery*, **21**(1), 93–98.

Migdal, C. (1994) Long-term functional outcome after early surgery in open-angle glaucoma. *Ophthalmology*, **101**(9), 1651–56.

Migdal, C. (1995) What is the appropriate treatment for patients with primary open-angle glaucoma: medicine, laser or primary surgery? *Ophthalmic Surgery*, **26**(2), 108–09.

National Service Framework for Diabetes (2002) Department of Health, London.

North, R. (2001) *Work and the Eye*, 2nd Edition. Oxford University Press, Oxford.

Nursing and Midwifery Council (2002) *Code of Professional Conduct*. DoH, HMSO, London.

O'Conner, S. and Glasper, E.A. (1995) *Whaley and Wong's Children's Nursing*. Mosby, London.

O'hEineachain, R. (2002) Cool Laser blasts way to micro-incision cataract surgery, www.escrs.org/eurotimes/December 2002/cool.asp

Osaka, M. and Keltuer, J. (1991) Botulinum A toxin (Oculinum) in ophthalmology. *Survey of Ophthalmology*, **36**(1), 28–46.

Ottar, W., Scott, W. and Holgado, S. (1995) Photoscreening for amblyogenic factors. *Journal of Pediatric Ophthalmology and Strabismus*, **32**, 289–95.

Patel, S. and Speath, G. (1995) Compliance in patients prescribed eye drops for glaucoma. *Ophthalmic Surgery*, **26**(3), 233–36.

Pearce, J. (1996) Multifocal intraocular lenses. *Current Opinion in Ophthalmology*, **7**(1), 2–10.

Potter, P.A. (1994) *Pocket Guide to Health Assessment*. Mosby, London.

Pratt-Johnson, J. and Tillson, G. (1994) *Management of Strasbismus and Amblyopia – A practical guide*. Theime Medical Publications Inc., New York.

Ragge, N. and Easty, D. (1990) *Immediate Eye Care*. Wolfe Publications, London.

Royal College of Ophthalmologists Guidelines (2002) Creutzfeldt-Jakob Disease (CJD) and Ophthalmology. http:www.site4sight.org.uk.

Rosen, A. and Knoop, D. (1982) Tolmectin-induced anaphylactoid reactions. *New England Journal of Medicine*, **307**, 499–500.

Saude, T. (1992) *Ocular Anatomy*. Blackwell Science, Oxford.

Schwab, I.R., Epstein, R.J., Harris, D.J., Pflugfelder, S.C., Wilhelmus, K.R. and Perry, P.E. (1997) External Eye Disease & Cornea.

Shaw, M. (2001) *Principles and Protocols for Ophthalmic Medication and Instillation/application* (In-house Policy), Manchester Royal Eye Hospital.

Sorsby, A. and Symons, H.M. (1946) Amniotic membrane grafts in caustic burns of the eye. *British Journal of Ophthalmology*, **30**, 337–45.

Stapleton, F. (1992) Microbial keratitis and contact lens wear. *Journal of British Contact Lens Association*, **3**(1), 5–6.

Szerenyi, K., Wang, X.W., Lee, M. and McDonnell, P.J. (1993) Topical diclofenac treatment prior to eximer laser photorefractive Keratometry in rabbits. *Refractive Corneal Surgery*, **9**, 437–42.

The Diabetes Control and Complications Trial Research Group (1995) The effect of intensive diabetes treatment on the progression of diabetic retinopathy in insulin dependent diabetes mellitus. *Archives of Ophthalmology*, **113**, 36–51.

Toma, N., Hungerford, J. and Plowman, P. et al. (1995) External beam radiotherapy for retinoblastoma 2-lens-sparing technique. *British Journal of Ophthalmology*, **79**(2), 112–17.

Tomask, R.L. (1997) *Handbook of treatment in neuro-ophthalmology.* Butterworth Heinemann, Boston.

Tsubota, K., Satake, Y. and Ohyama, M. (1996) Surgical reconstruction of the ocular surface in advanced ocular cicatricial pemphigoid and Stevens Johnson syndrome. *American Journal of Ophthalmology,* **122,** 38–52.

Vaughan, D., Asbury, T. and Riordan-Eva, P. (1999) *General Ophthalmology.* Lange Medical Publications, New York.

Visto, D. (2000) Corneal abrasion: To patch or not to patch. *Insight,* 25, Jan–March.

Wakelin, S. (1995) Hygiene compliance in contact lens wearers presenting to an ophthalmic casualty department. *The International Journal of Pharmacy Practice,* **3**(2), 97–100.

Waterman, H., Leatherbarrow, B.L., Waterman, C. and Hillier, V. (1998) Postoperative nausea and vomiting following hydroxyapatite orbital implant. *European Journal of Anaesthesiology,* **15,** 590–94.

Williams, M. (1993) Achieving patient compliance. *Nursing Times,* **89**(13), 50–52.

Wilson, C.G. and O'Mahoney, B. (1999) Non-compliance in glaucoma management *Eyenews,* **5**(6), 7–9.

Wittpen, J.R. (1995) Eye Scrub: Simplifying the management of blepharitis. *Journal of Ophthalmic Nursing & Technology,* **14**(1), 25–28.

Yung, C.W., Massicotte, S. and Kuwabara, T. (1994) Argon laser treatment of trichiasis – a clinical and histopathologic evaluation. *Ophthalmic Plastic Reconstructive Surgery,* **10**(2), 130–36.

Websites of interest

http://www.gpnotebook.co.uk Compliance with medication.
http://www.brit-thoracic.org.uk
http://www.bham.ac.uk/arif/odonto.htm
http://www.wihrd.soton.ac.uk/projx/signpost/steers/STEER_2001(6)_APRX.pdf
http://bjo.bmjjournals.com/cgi/content/abstract/76/4/232

Index

Page numbers in *italics* refer to Colour Plates